Eye Surgery

Eye Surgery

Edited by Eleanor McCarthy

hayle medical

New York

Hayle Medical,
750 Third Avenue, 9th Floor,
New York, NY 10017, USA

Visit us on the World Wide Web at:
www.haylemedical.com

ISBN: 978-1-63241-705-3

Cataloging-in-Publication Data

Eye surgery / edited by Eleanor McCarthy.
    p. cm.
Includes bibliographical references and index.
ISBN 978-1-63241-705-3
1. Eye--Surgery. 2. Eye--Surgery--Complications. 3. Eye--Diseases.
I. McCarthy, Eleanor.
RE80 .E94 2019
617.71--dc23

Table of Contents

Preface

Eye surgery or ocular surgery is the surgery performed on the eye or its adnexa, including the eyebrows, eyelids and lacrimal apparatus. It is a sensitive procedure requiring extreme care, before, during and after the procedure to prevent or minimize any damage. Conditions of the eye, such as myopia, hypermetropia and astigmatism can be addressed through a laser eye surgery. Cataract surgery is a widely practiced type of eye surgery. It is performed to correct any opacification or cloudiness of the eye lens. Other common procedures such as refractive surgery, vitreo-retinal surgery, corneal surgery, oculoplastic surgery, etc. are performed to treat abnormalities in the eye. Due to the dense network of nerves in the eye, ocular surgery is always performed under anesthesia, whether local, topical or general. This book is a valuable compilation of topics, ranging from the basic to the most complex advancements in the field of eye surgery. It presents this complex subject in the most comprehensible language. It is a vital tool for all researching or studying ocular surgery and ophthalmology, as it gives incredible insights into emerging trends and concepts.

All of the data presented henceforth, was collaborated in the wake of recent advancements in the field. The aim of this book is to present the diversified developments from across the globe in a comprehensible manner. The opinions expressed in each chapter belong solely to the contributing authors. Their interpretations of the topics are the integral part of this book, which I have carefully compiled for a better understanding of the readers.

At the end, I would like to thank all those who dedicated their time and efforts for the successful completion of this book. I also wish to convey my gratitude towards my friends and family who supported me at every step.

Editor

Cataract Surgery

Sanja Masnec and Miro Kalauz

Abstract

Phacoemulsification is the most common ophthalmic surgery and it revolutionized cataract surgery. With the introduction of sutureless clear corneal incisions surgical time has been reduced, faster postoperative recovery enabled, and induced astigmatism lowered. Various premium intraocular lenses (IOLs) such as multifocal, accommodative and toric IOLs are designed to enable the best refractive outcomes. In order to further increase accuracy and precision femtosecond laser assisted cataract surgery (FLACS) has been introduced with ability to perform incisions, capsulorhexis and disassembly of the lens.

Most frequent long-term complication of cataract surgery is posterior capsule opacification (PCO). Another most common cause of patient dissatisfaction after uneventful surgery is pseudophakic dysphotopsia. Acrylic materials with a higher index of refraction and square edge designed IOLs are developed in order to minimise PCO, but on the other hand they seem to enhance dysphotopic phenomena in patients.

To achieve the best possible postoperative result, careful selection of patients, individual approach and patient education is mandatory.

Keywords: Phacoemulsification, clear corneal incision, intraocular lens, posterior capsule opacification, pseudophakic dysphotopsia

1. Introduction

Cataract surgery is the most common ophthalmic surgery, and one of the most frequently performed surgeries in general. A "cataract" refers to a focal or diffuse opacification of the crystalline lens, a structure that is normally opticaly clear. Hardening and clouding of the lens may result in a progressive loss of vision depending on its size, location and density. It is typically bilateral, compromises visual acuity and contrast sensitivity and increases glare. Cataract may form at any age due to a number of different etiologies such as systemic metabolic disease, use of different medications, ocular trauma, but most often is age related. As the lens ages, it increases in weight and thickness and decreases in accommodative power. In cross-sectional studies, the prevalence of cataracts is 50% in people between the ages of 65 and 74 and it increases to 70% in those over the age of 75 [1]. The pathogenesis of age-related cataracts is multifactorial and not completely understood. Different methods have been developed for cataract surgery, such as intracapsular and extracapsular extraction procedures, but the most common and widely accepted procedure is phacoemulsification, since its development in 1967, by Charles Kelman [2].

2. Phacoemulsification

The procedure of phacoemulsification has gained increasing popularity worldwide, since the introduction of sutureless clear corneal cataract incisions, due to several advantages over the traditional sutured scleral tunnels and limbal incisions [3]. Several surgical approaches have been suggested to allow for a faster and easier phacoemulsification technique. The introduction of clear corneal incisions to enter the anterior chamber and remove the cataract using phacoemulsification revolutionized cataract surgery [4]. This approach is the most popular and widely accepted. Clear corneal wounds have transformed cataract surgery by dramatically reducing surgical time, offering faster postoperative recovery, and lowering the induced astigmatism in comparison to scleral tunnel incisions [3].

3. Scleral tunnel incisions

Scleral incisions in phacoemulsification were firstly introduced by Girard and Hoffman [5]. The incision size is usually 3-7 mm in chord length [6]. Smaller incisions may be sutureless while larger tunnels often are sutured and periotomy is performed in both cases. Scleral tunnel construction could lead to several problems. An initial scleral tunnel that is too deep will create scleral disinsertion with exposure to the ciliary body leading to different problems with hemostasis, poor wound stability, early or posterior entry to the anterior chamber, and iris prolapse. On the other hand, an incision that is too shallow may result in tear of the tunnel roof and problems with water tightness of the wound [3]. Another thing that is of great importance is the length of scleral tunnel. A dissection that is too far into the cornea creates an anterior entry into the anterior chamber resulting in decreased maneuverability and corneal striae that interfere with visibility during subsequent steps. An incision that is too short would create problems with wound closure and iris prolapse [3]. Other complicaions include induced astigmatism, filtration, hyphema and Descemets membrane detachment.

4. Limbal incisions

The differences in the healing effects of incisions at the limbus and the cornea are widely discussed in the literature [7-9]. Limbal incisions are likely to heal more quickly and are more resistant to deformation pressure than those in the cornea. Reasons for that are significant anatomical and physiological differences between them. Regular lamellar structure of collagen fibrils of the cornea stretch from limbus to limbus. It is arranged in a lattice formation and provides the primary structural support of the cornea and its transparency. The cornea is avascular.

On the other hand, at the limbus, this regular structure is no longer present. Vascular arcades are evident, providing a potential source of fibroblasts [10] in the effects of clear corneal and scleral or limbal incisions, related to differences in the respective structures where the incisions are made.

In comparison to limbal incisions, clear corneal incisions also appear to increase the likelihood of endophthalmitis [11, 12].

5. Clear Corneal Incisions (CCIs)

Sutureless clear corneal incisions are the most common incisions for cataract surgery with phacoemulsification, replacing scleral tunnel and limbal incisions. There are several reasons for the popularity of clear corneal approach based on different advantages compared to scleral tunnel incisions. Some of them include reduced procedure time, lower induced astigmatism, faster visual recovery and less complications.

The aim of cataract surgery today is rapid visual rehabilitation, the best possible uncorrected visual acuity, and minimal postoperative astigmatism. The phacoemulsification procedure results in less surgically induced astigmatism than extracapsular cataract extraction, in which the incision is much larger. Clear corneal incision is the most used type of incision in phacoemulsification surgery, because it is less time-consuming and does not require cauterization or wound suturing. The location of the CCI affects the degree of postoperative astigmatism. One of the possible complications of cataract surgery is surgically induced astigmatism (SIA), which is a major cause of functional disturbance and insufficient uncorrected visual acuity. CCI is made deliberately in the steepest meridian if astigmatism is addressed. It can be made at superior, oblique or temporal locations. Temporal CCI induces regular astigmatism 90 degrees away from the incision (with-the-rule astigmatism) thus minimizing the postoperative astigmatism [13-15]. It is known to induce the least postoperative astigmatism. Also, the smaller the CCI, the lesser the induced astigmatism. Oblique scleral tunnel incision predictably reduces astigmatism by simultaneously producing corneal flattening and steepening [16].

Some studies have shown that a small superior CCI induces greater postoperative astigmatism than a small supero-oblique CCI, and a small supero-oblique CCI induces higher postoperative astigmatism than a small temporal CCI [17-19]. Some authors reported that, although temporal

CCI is reported to result in the least induced astigmatism, locating the incision superotemporally or superonasally may ease surgical manipulations during the phacoemulsification cataract surgery for a right-handed surgeon who works from the 12 o'clock position relative to the patient [20]. Performing the procedure from the patient's temporal side may not be possible with the most operating tables, and locating the CCI temporally in the left eye may be difficult for a right-handed surgeon who sits at the 12 o'clock position.

Several groups of authors analyzed refractive astigmatism in patients who have had phacoemulsification cataract surgery performed by the oblique clear corneal incision. They provided evidence that the supero-oblique clear corneal incision does not induce the clinically significant amount of oblique astigmatism [21-23]. Also, evidence is provided that the superotemporal or superonasal CCI has minimal effect on corneal astigmatism [23]. Many studies investigated the influence of different factors, such as the type of a surgery, length of incision and its type (curved, straight, frown), location and width of incision (central vs. peripheral-limbal or scleral), presence or absence of a suture and the suturing method, on postoperative astigmatism [16, 19, 24, 25]. Any incisions that are made in the cornea have the potential to change the curvature and therefore the dioptric power of the cornea in that meridian. The location as well as the width of the incision affects the degree of postoperative astigmatism.Surgically induced astigmatism is positively correlated with incision size (larger incisions generating more astigmatism) and location (scleral or limbal incision inducing less astigmatism than clear corneal), though for small incisions the effect of location appears less critical [26, 27]. Wound construction also appears to have an effect, with square incisions reported to affect astigmatism the least [28]. Despite all the advantages of clear corneal incisions, they are not without problems. Reported disadvantages include poor wound healing [29], induction of irregular astigmatism [29], the risk of wound dehiscence following trivial trauma [30], and increased loss of endothelial cells [31].

5.1. Overview of the technique

Phacoemulsification in most cases begins with a 2.2 to 3.0 mm tunnel in the peripheral corneal to enter to the anterior chamber. Reduced incision size to 2.2 mm and smaller led to several innovations in instrumentation, phacoemulsification technology, and intraocular lens (IOL) design. Each step taken in reducing the incision size comes with mixed success but has led ultimately to measurable improvements in outcomes [32]. During intraocular surgery, the anterior chamber is stabilized with an ophthalmic viscoelastic device (OVD).Continuous curvilinear capsulorhexis is made at the anterior surface of the lens capsule, followed by hydrodissection that separates the capsule and cortex and hydro-delineation that separates the nucleus from epinucleus and cortex (in cases of medium or medium-hard nucleus). Phacoemulsification begins when the tip of a handpiece connected to the phaco machine is placed within the anterior chamber to fracture the lens into the small pieces and to aspirate the remaining small particles. Aspiration uses pumping to remove liquid and debris generated during the surgery. Pumping creates a partial vacuum and the negative pressure forces liquid out. To maintain the anterior chamber volume, irrigation of the saline-like solution is performed at the same time. After fragmentation and aspiration, insertion of the artificial intraocular foldable lens via injector follows. Continuous longitudinal ultrasound (US) has an inherent repulsive characteristic that can induce turbulence, cause chatter, and create substantial heat along the shaft of the phaco needle. Larger bore needles allow greater fluid flow allowing better cooling and transfer of larger fragments of nuclear material. Fortunately, none of the current generation phaco units rely solely on continuous longitudinal power [32]. Micropulse phacoemulsification is a result of advancements in phacoemulsification modalities that include less power use and shorter procedure times. The operating temperature of the needle in the incision is decreased [33, 34]. The next progression provided torsional phacoemulsification (Ozil, Alcon Laboratories, Inc.) with needle temperature also reduced [35]. Transversal phacoemulsification (Ellips, Abbott Medical Optics, Inc.), the next nonlongitudinal movement, has a similar effect. Each of these power modulations has resulted in improved ultrasonic efficiency and can use smaller gauge needles to effectively emulsify nuclear material [32].

6. Phacodynamics

Modern phacoemulsification machines generate the required vacuum and aspiration based on one of three pumping systems:

1. Peristaltic pump

2. Venturi pump

3. Diaphragm pump

1. Peristaltic pump

In this type of pump, the fluid is displaced through flexible tubing using a series of rollers on a rotating wheel. As the wheel rotates, the rollers move the fluid trapped between them, which result in more fluid being drawn into the tubing in the direction of rotation (Figure 1). The flow rate is directly proportional to the speed of the rotary mechanism. At low speeds of rotation a vacuum is not produced unless the tip is occluded. As the speed of rotation is increased, a vacuum is produced in the aspiration line without occlusion. A desired flow rate and vacuum is determined by the surgeon.

2. Venturi pump

There is no moving part in this pump. This type of pump works on Bernoulli's principle. When the speed of flow of a fluid is increased in one part, the pressure in that part is decreased. Compressed gas, such as air or nitrogen, flowing through a pipe (Figure 2) reduces the pressure in the next region and creates a partial vacuum within the rigid drainage cassette.

3. Diaphragm pump

In this type of pump, a flexible metal or rubber diaphragm moves up and down. This movement, along with the vertical motion of two valves, maintains the vacuum (Figure 3). Clinically, this type of pump is similar to the Venturi pump.

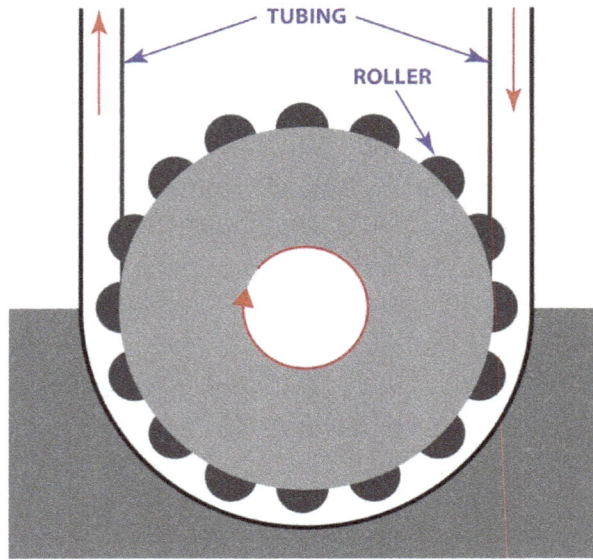

Figure 1. Peristaltic pump

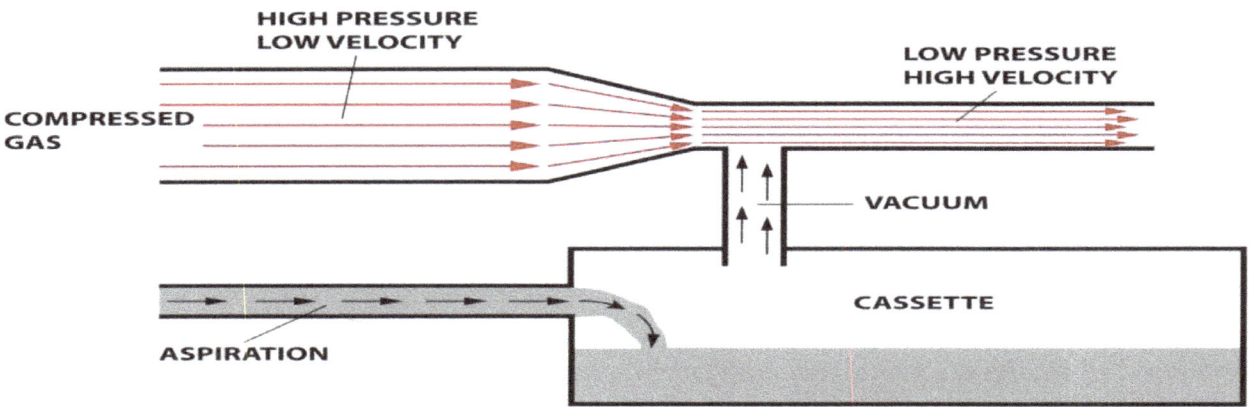

Figure 2. Venturi pump

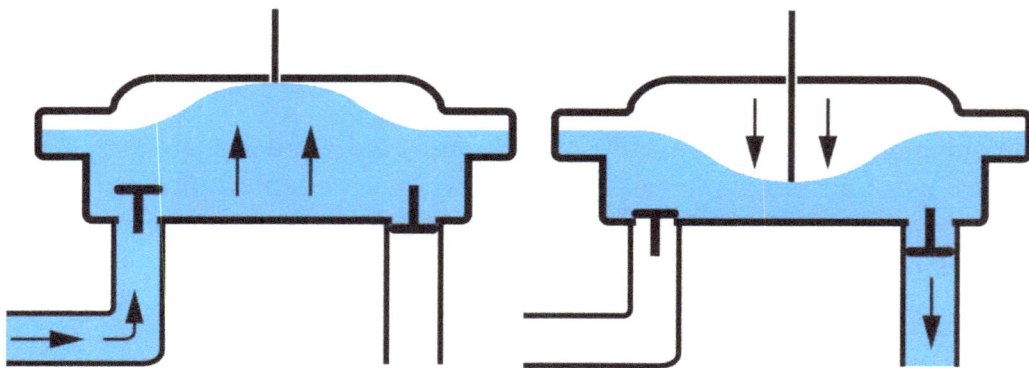

Figure 3. Diaphragm pump

The peristaltic pump has a slower rise time unlike the Venturi and diaphragm pumps that have rapid flow rates and rise times. Rise time measures how rapidly a vacuum builds up once occlusion has occured at the aspiration tip. Flow rate measures the amount of fluid passing through the tubing (cc/min) and indicates how quickly events will progress once the aspiration tip is either suddenly occluded or suddenly cleared. Venturi and diaphragm pumps have higher flow rates and therefore they build up vacuums in the aspirate line without occlusion of the aspiration tip. Once the tip is occluded, a vacuum builds up rapidly [2, 36-38].

Peristaltic	Venturi
Flow based	Vacuum based
Vacuum created on occlusion of phaco tip	Vacuum created instantly via pump
Flow is constant until occlusion	Flow varies with vacuum level
Drains into a soft bag	Drains into a rigid cassette

Table 1. Differences between pumps, as reported by Devgan [38].

7. Intraocular Lenses (IOLs)

Nowadays, cataract surgery is not synonymous with lens extraction; it evolved in a more refined procedure due to advances in phacoemulsification procedure and intraocular lens technology [39]. The most frequent and the cheapest intraocular lenses are monofocal. After their implantation most patients need spectacles, at least for near vision. The goal of premium IOL design is to enable the best refractive outcome with restoration of vision for distance and near without spectacles. Multifocal and accommodative intraocular lenses, as well as toric IOLs for corneal astigmatism compensation, are considered premium IOLs. The aim of multifocal and accommodative premium IOLs is to allow the presbyopic patient to regain the ability to accommodate. The capacity of the eye to actively change its refractive power to create a sharp image on the retina of distant, intermediate, and near objects is called accommodation [40].

7.1. Multifocal IOLs

Multifocal IOLs focus light in more than one point. They are described as refractive, diffractive, and combinations of both optical principles. Also, they can be spherical and aspherical. They were first introduced in the 1980s [41, 42]. They consist of multiple circular, concentric areas that provide a continuous variation of the refractive power. Diffractive multifocal artificial lenses are based on the HuygensFresnel principle [43] presenting concentric rings that result in two or more coexisting retinal images and are independent of pupil size.

On the other hand, refractive IOLs are dependent on pupil size. Refraction is based on a change in direction of the light ray due to a change in the optical density of the material transmitting the light ray. Refractive IOLs provide usually good near vision but are mostly insufficient regarding very small prints [44]. Recent studies report very good results in most cases after implantation of a multifocal IOL, diffractive [45-47], refractive [46, 47], or hybrid diffractive-refractive [48]. Aspheric multifocals decrease higher-order aberrations of the ocular optical system, primarily by compensating for the increased positive spherical aberration of the cornea in older subjects [49, 50].They provide a significantly better near visual acuity compared to spherical multifocal IOLs, with no significant influence on night vision symptoms and contrast sensitivity [51]. Various studies have shown that uncorrected near vision is improved by implantation of a multifocal IOL in comparison to monofocal IOL, resulting in lower levels of spectacle dependence for near tasks without compromising distance visual acuity [52-58]. In general, multifocal IOLs are able to provide patients with excellent uncorrected distance and near visual acuity resulting in high levels of spectacle independence [49]. Although, the preceding discussion makes the multifocals very appealing, they are not devoid of problems. One of the main reasons for patient dissatisfaction is dysphotopsia [59, 60]. The most reported phenomena after multifocal IOL implantation are halos and glare [61, 62], especially in refractive multifocal IOLs [46]. In general, multifocal IOLs are associated with lower contrast sensitivity than monofocal IOLs [46]. Regarding that, diffractive multifocal IOLs appear to be equal or superior to refractive multifocal IOLs [63, 64]. Also, multifocal IOLs have been associated with higher levels of high order aberrations (HOAs) than monofocal IOLs [65]. Refractive multifocal IOLs performed better at intermediate than near distance [51, 66]. Diffractive multifocal IOLs with lower near additions have increased visual acuity at inter-mediate distance without decreasing near and distance visual acuity [48, 67]. Lately, it has been shown that intermediate visual acuity is increased with trifocal diffractive IOLs [68]. In preoperative evaluation, it is of great importance careful selection of patients, individual approach, patient s education and consideration of all benefits and side-effects of multifocal IOLs [69, 70].

7.2. Accommodative IOLs

An alternative to multifocal lenses are accommodative lenses, which are able to change position or shape in response to the accommodative reflex. They were designed to avoid the optical side effects of multifocal IOLs and to offer the best solution for presbyopia: an IOL of high-amplitude variable focality [71]. They are classified according to design into single-optic, dual-optic, and curvature change IOLs [72]. Accommodative lenses act like monofocal lenses, but provide better visual acuity for intermediate and distance vision. In comparison to multifocals, they are independent on pupil size and therefore provide less disphotopic effects and do not decrease contrast sensitivity. On the other hand, there is a variability of the postoperative outcome, greater risk for capsular contraction and opacification, and the need for further near vision correction [73]. Ideal IOL would allow the presbyopic patient to regain his or her ability to accommodate. Experiments have been conducted with refilling the capsular bag with a clear and elastic substance in order to achieve desirable accommodation, but unfortunately unsuccessfuly [74]. Also, different attempts with the change in position of the IOL or parts of it within the optical system in order to change the optical power of the optical system and to restore the patient's accommodation in that way have not resulted as expected [75]. Some of the ultrasound studies showed changes in the position of accommodating IOLs within the optical system in response to physiological or pharmaceutical stimuli [76], while others did not provide evidence of significant movement of those IOLs [77, 78]. Looking into a clinical practice, accommodating IOLs seems to be insufficient to result in large changes in the power of the optical system [75, 79].

7.3. Toric IOLs

Approximately 20% to 30% of patients who have cataract surgery have corneal astigmatism of 1.25 diopters (D) or higher and approximately 10% of patients have 2.00 D or higher [80-82]. Toric intraocular lenses are a predictable method of astigmatic correction with minimal impact to the cornea. Based on current evidence, it appears that a minimal amount of corneal astigmatism of approximately 1.25 D should be present before toric IOL implantation is considered [83]. They provide an opportunity for corneal astigmatism correction at the time of cataract surgery and for spectacle independence. But, effectiveness of torics is dependent on its orientation [84, 85]. A 10-degree error in rotation results in a 35% residual error in the magnitude of astigmatism. Since the beginning of the first implanted foldable toric intraocular lens in 1994 [86-89], many improvements in IOL material and design have been made to improve postoperative rotational stability and therefore improved visual outcomes following toric IOL implantation. Toric IOLs are made of hydrophobic acrylic, hydrophilic acrylic, silicone, or polymethylmethacrylate (PMMA) biomaterial. The IOL biomaterial plays a major role in the postoperative rotation of the IOL. After implantation of a toric IOL in the capsular bag, the anterior and posterior capsules fuse with the IOL, preventing IOL rotation [90]. Adhesions of the IOL to the capsular bag are thought to prevent IOL rotation. Lombardo et al. found that hydrophobic acrylic IOLs showed the highest adhesive properties, followed by hydrophilic acrylic IOLs, PMMA IOLs, and finally silicone IOLs [91]. Oshika et al. showed the strongest IOL–capsular bag adhesions for acrylic IOLs, followed by PMMA and silicone IOLs [92]. Acrylic IOLs generally form the strongest adhesions with the capsular bag [90]. Also, IOL design contributes to the stability of the lens in the capsular bag and avoidance of postoperative IOL rotation. It has been shown that the overall IOL diameter and haptic design are major factors in the prevention of IOL rotation [93-95]. Currently available toric IOLs have a total IOL diameter ranging from 11.0 mm to 13.0 mm. The lens with longer IOL diameter was found to have much better rotational stability than the lens with shorter diameter [94]. Two haptic designs are available: plate-haptic and loop-haptic. When comparing the postoperative rotation of plate versus loop-haptic silicone IOLs, some studies found significantly higher postoperative rotation with loop-haptic IOLs than with plate-haptic IOLs [93]. Others compared plate-haptic and loop-haptic acrylic IOLs and did not find a significant difference in postoperative rotation, suggesting that in acrylic IOLs, plate and loop haptics have both good rotational stability [96]. Toric IOLs are most effective in the correction of regular astigmatism, but they have been shown to be effective in patients with irregular corneal astigmatism, including keratoconus (only if the risk for progression is minimal) [97], pellucid marginal degeneration [98], and post-keratoplasty eyes [99, 100]. Not suitable for torics are patients with potential capsular bag instability, like those with pseudoexfoliation syndrome or trauma-induced zonulysis because zonular weakness affects IOL stability and may result in rotation or decentration of a toric IOL [83]. Multifocal toric IOLs gain for spectacle independence regarding distance, intermediate, and near vision. Evidence has been provided that the presence of 1.00 D or higher astigmatism in eyes with a multifocal IOL compromise distance and near visual acuity, showing the importance of an optimal astigmatism correction in these patients [101].

8. Complications

8.1. Posterior capsular opacification (PCO)

The most frequent long-term complication of cataract surgery remains posterior capsule opacification (PCO), an after cataract. In the past two decades, refinements in surgical technique and modifications in intraocular lens (IOL) design and material have led to a decrease in the incidence of PCO [102]. Symptoms of posterior capsule opacification include blurred vision and are similar to those of a normal cataract. Patients may also see streaks of light, halos, or excessive glare.

It has been shown that a sharp posterior optic edge inhibits migration of lens epithelial cells (LECs) behind the IOL optic and results in a lower incidence of PCO [103-106]. Most IOL designs, especially multipiece, have open-loop haptics that have a relatively narrow optic–haptic junction. The junction is thought to be an Achilles heel for LEC migration, and the narrower the junction, the better the optic-edge effect against LEC migration [106].

As intraocular lens (IOL) design [107, 108], the material [91, 109, 110], and the surgical technique [111, 112] play a crucial role in retarding the development of central posterior capsule opacification (PCO). Intraocular lens materials can be broadly divided into hydrophobic and hydrophilic based on their surface energy. Acrylic IOLs with a hydrophobic or hydrophilic surface are widely used in practice [113, 114].Single-piece hydrophilic acrylic IOLs with a modified square edge are also available. The PCO rate with these hydrophilic IOLs, which have an improved 360-degree sharp edge, is reportedly lower than with older hydrophilic models that had a sharp optic edge design except at the optic–haptic junction [115].

Studies [113, 116] have compared PCO between older hydrophilic IOL models and single-piece hydrophobic acrylic IOLs, with the results favoring the latter. Because IOL characteristics play a crucial role in preventing PCO, it is important to assess PCO formation after implantation of these IOLs. This would help clinicians and researchers understand the impact of IOL material and design on the development of PCO.

Several studies report low PCO rates with square-edged IOLs and increased PCO with hydrophilic IOLs [117, 118]. However, both IOL material and design are important factors in the development of PCO.

The mechanism of action is hypothetically caused by a mechanical barrier effect of a sharp optic edge [106], by contact inhibition of the migrating LECs at the capsular bend by the square edge [107], and/or by the high pressure exerted by IOLs with a square-edged optic profile on the posterior capsule bend [108]. Based on these findings, various IOLs with often only minor differences in material and design were launched. With the introduction of 1-piece (monobloc)

IOL designs, which are easier to implant and to manufacture, there was concern about a loss of the barrier effect to the migration of LECs in the region of the optic–haptic junction. The broad-based bulky haptics of 1-piece IOLs extending from the optic rim inherently interfere with capsular bag fusion, thus bending the posterior capsule. However, comparing 1- and 3-piece Acrysof IOLs, no statistically significant difference in PCO was found in the long run [103]. A study comparing two models of 1-piece hydrophilic acrylic IOLs showed significantly less PCO in the eyes with an IOL with a square edge across the optic–haptic junction than matched eyes with an IOL without a square edge at the junction 1 year after surgery [117]. For the most part, a square posterior optic edge has been considered the major factor in the prevention of PCO formation. Hydrophobic acrylic IOLs are not manufactured from the same materials or by using the same processes. Therefore, the polymers used differ in their chemical structure, water content, and refractive indices. Material differences are also reflected by the tendency toward glistening formation. Microvacuoles within the IOL material can occur when the IOL is in an aqueous environment and water fills microscopic openings in the material. Typical with acrylic IOLs, glistenings appear as white sparkling areas over the entire IOL optic, which may impair the optical quality. The higher density of the acrylic polymer network may prevent the formation of microvacuoles and provide better visual outcomes. Several studies conclude that hydrophobic IOLs are better than hydrophilic IOLs in preventing PCO [113, 116, 117].However, most comparisons have been between hydrophilic IOLs with round edges and hydrophobic IOLs with sharp edges.Regarding IOL design, the theory that an IOL with a sharp posterior optic edge prevents PCO has gained acceptance. There are two theories of how a sharp-edged optic inhibits PCO formation [103-105]. One is the compression theory, which suggests that contact pressure between the posterior capsule and the IOL optic edge mechanically prevents cell migration[103]. The other is that a sharp optic edge induces the formation of a sharp capsular bend, which creates contact inhibition between migrating lens epithelial cells (LECs) [104, 105]. Experimental and clinical studies suggest that the sharper the capsular bend, the greater the preventive effect [106]. Analysis of the microstructure of the optic edge of currently available square-edged hydrophilic and hydrophobic acrylic IOLs showed a large variation in the deviation from a perfect square, not only between IOL designs but also between different powers of the same IOL design.

The optic–haptic junction is another important factor in preventing PCO. In one study [105], eyes with an IOL with a continuous 360-degree square edge had significantly less PCO than eyes with an IOL with a square edge that was interrupted at the optic–haptic junction. Accordingly, it is hard to say which IOL has a proper design in terms of preventing PCO. It would be ideal for clinical PCO comparison studies to evaluate IOLs with the same material or design, although this would be difficult using currently available IOLs.

There are few studies comparing hydrophilic IOLs with a sharp edge and hydrophobic IOLs with a sharp edge [109, 113, 116]. In a study with a 2-year follow-up, Kugelberg et al. [109] found that patients with the Acrysof SA60AT hydrophobic acrylic IOL had less PCO than patients with the BL27 hydrophilic acrylic IOL (Bausch & Lomb). Others found no significant differences in the PCO and Nd:YAG rates between the hydrophobic group and hydrophilic group 3 years after surgery [113, 116].

Animal [119] and clinical [108] studies show that IOL design, rather than IOL material, is the critical factor in minimizing LEC migration across the posterior capsule after IOL implantation. The continuous-edge IOL has two design characteristics that may have led to the significant decrease in PCO, and that is a 360-degree continuous square optic edge, and greater space between the optic and haptic at the optic–haptic junction to encourage apposition of the anterior capsule and posterior capsule. A continuous square edge around the optic and angled haptics allows close apposition of the IOL optic to the posterior capsule, which Nishi et al. [120] found inhibits LEC migration. A rabbit model study [121] found that the addition of a square edge across the optic–haptic junction decreased LEC migration behind the IOL optic over migration with an IOL of the same type but without a square edge at the optic–haptic junction.

In the treatment of PCO, neodymium: yttrium-aluminum-garnet (ND:YAG) laser is used to cut the clouded posterior capsule allowing light to transmit normally [122]. It can produce complications such as ocular inflammation, an increase in intraocular pressure, IOL damage, cystoid macular edema, and retinal detachment.

9. Pseudophakic dysphotopsia

One of the most common causes of patient dissatisfaction after uneventful cataract surgery is a pseudophakic dysphotopsia [123, 124]. It represents a set of subjective optical complaints following intraocular lens implantation and is categorized as positive and negative dysphotopsia. Positive dysphotopsia are bright artifacts on the retina that represent undesired optical images described by the patients as halos, arcs, light rings, flashes, and streaks. The phenomenon called negative dysphotopsia manifests as a temporal dark crescent-shaped shadow, similar to scotoma, and represents the absence of light reaching certain portions of the retina after in the-bag posterior chamber IOL implantation [125]. It has been first described almost 15 years ago, by Davison [126] and since then it is a matter of discussion in many scientific papers. The cause of this phenomena has been widely discussed in the literature and many explanations have been proposed such as optics with a sharp or truncated edge [124, 126, 127], IOL materials with high index of refraction [126-130], anatomical predispositions of the eye such as prominent globe [131], shallow orbit [131], anterior surface of the IOL more then 0.46 mm from the plane of posterior iris [131], brown iris [132], temporally located clear cornea incisions [132], a negative afterimage [133], neuroadaptation [133], and reflection of the anterior capsulotomy edge projected onto the nasal peripheral retina [134]. Negative dysphotopsia is more poorly tolerated than positive and could lead to IOL explantation [131, 135, 136]. Certain clinical manifestations have been recognized and nicely summarized by Masket and Fram [134].

Still, there has not been much theoretical exploration in the past to explain in detail and to validate all possible explanations of the negative dysphotopsia phenomenon. In the recent study, designed to evaluate negative dysphotopsia, Holladay et al. [125] used ray tracing simulation, using the Zemax optical design program and described "type 3 shadow-penumbra" as the optical mechanism that has been referred to as negative dysphotopsia and believe that it explains all 10 clinical manifestations enumerated by Masket and Fram [134].They concluded that primary optical factors for negative dyshotopsia are small pupil, a distance behind the pupil of ≥0.06 mm and ≤ 1.23 mm for acrylic (≥ 0.06 mm and ≤ 0.62 mm for silicone), a sharp-edged design (corner edge radii ≤ 0.05 mm) and functional nasal retina that extends anterior to the location of the shadow. The final parameter that determines whether the shadow is visible is the location of the anterior extent of the functional nasal retina. Secondary factors include the high index of refraction optic material, the patient's angle α, nasal location of the pupil relative to the optical axis, and transparent versus translucent status of the peripheral nasal capsule [125].

Holladay et al. showed that a sharp or truncated optic edge was the most significant factor in positive dysphotopsia[124].Advances in lens edge design have minimized such problems, but still a significant number of patients report of different photic phenomena [123, 124, 127, 137]. Square-edge IOL design appears to be the primary cause of reflected nighttime glare [124]. Radford et al. reported on overall incidence of 20.7% in the Akreos group and 21.3% in the SN60-AT group [127]. Also, a study of patient-reported glare symptoms found fewer symptoms with Akreos IOLs than with other acrylic lenses [138]. Osher reported the incidence of negative dysphotopsia 15.2% on the first postoperative day, decreasing to 3.2% after 1 year, then 2.4% after 2 and 3 years. Kinard et al. reported on 40% of study patients complaining about central flashes 1 year postoperatively, and 3% rating it with the highest score. They found that some of the patients originally thought to be a complete success had dissatisfaction from dysphotopsia but silently put up with it [139]. The mechanism of neuroadaptation is still the least understood of all factors involved in the process of pseudophakic dysphotopsia. As Jin et al. disscussed, there are patients who have 2-mm IOL dislocation who should have debilitating dysphotopsia and yet adapt very nicely. On the other hand, some have perfectly centred IOL with excellent vision, good coverage of the IOL edge by the anterior capsule, and still report severe symptoms of dysphotopsia long after surgery [137]. Holladay said that neural adaptation can mitigate and reduce symptoms but not eliminate them, just as halos with multifocal IOLs diminish with time but never disappear [140]. The positive symptoms seem to diminish with time, or the patients get more used to them. Regarding the IOL features that could contribute to dysphotopsia, hydrophobic acrylic lenses with higher refractive index have a greater risk of dysphotopsia [126-130]. On the other hand, hydrophilic acrylic intraocular lenses with lower refractive index could be superior in that matter due to less affinity toward dysphotopsia [126-130]. Bournas et al. showed that the lens optic diameter is negatively associated with the risk of dysphotopsia [141]. It is believed that with 6.0 mm, 6.5 mm, and 7.0 mm intraocular lenses are less likely to experience the photic phenomena because the edge line of the IOL is out of view [142, 143]. On the other hand, Arnold concluded that the optic size of the IOL does not correlate with any forms of dysphotopsia [144]. Four surgical methods were used to treat negative dysphotopsia: secondary piggyback IOL implantation, reverse optic capture, in-the-bag exchange, and iris suture fixation [131, 134, 136, 145]. Holladay explained that exchanging the posterior chamber IOL for an anterior chamber IOL or using a fully (not partially) rounded-edge IOL are the only two treatments that are sure to eliminate negative dysphotopsia. Exchanges for a silicone material, secondary piggyback IOLs, and reverse optic capture usually will improve the symptoms but cannot guarantee elimination of negative dysphotopsia [140]. Folden recently presented a Neodymium:Yag laser anterior capsulectomy as a surgical option in the management of negative dysphotopsia [146]. Osher believed that short term, transient symptoms of negative dysphotopsia were incision related, mostly at patients with clear temporal incision, were the cornea is not covered by the eyelid. He hypothesized that corneal edema-associated beveled temporal incision was related to the transient symptoms of dysphotopsia [132]. On the other hand, Cooke described a case where negative dysphotopsia resolved after IOL exchange with clear temporal incision, after prior surgery with scleral tunnel incision at 10.30 o'clock position, entirely covered by the upper lid [147]. Radford et al. stated that although 22% of patients who had a clear temporal incision and 66% of patients who had a superior scleral incision reported symptoms of dysphotopsia at 1 week, the difference between groups was not statistically significant. At 8 weeks 16% of patients with a clear temporal incision and 42% of patients with superior scleral incision reported symptoms of dysphotopsia, however the difference was not statistically significant again [127]. Also, additional studies comparing temporal clear corneal incisions with nasal [128] and superior [131] found no difference in the incidence of negative dysphotopsia. Although a significant number of patients report photic phenomena, it seems to resolve over time in the majority of cases [141, 144, 148]. They resolve by capsule opacification due to fibrosis, cortical adaptation, or a patients final compromise with the problem [149]. It is important to consider the amount of time between the surgery and telephone contact date because as time goes by, anterior capsule opacification (ACO) may shield the optic edge from light, protecting the patient from edge effects [150]. Holladay et al. agree with Hong et al.[151] that the spontaneous resolution or transient nature of negative dysphotopsia is a result of opacification (translucency/diffusivity) of the peripheral capsule. They stated that the opacification of the nasal capsule is the explanation for 12.8% of negative dysphotopsia that spontaneously resolved by 2 or 3 years of the original 15.2% in Osher's study [125], mentioned earlier.

10. Femtosecond Laser Assisted Cataract Surgery (FLACS)

Since premium intraocular lenses (IOLs) are getting more used for the achievement of the best refractive outcome, methods to increase accuracy and precision in cataract surgery are being investigated [152-154]. Femtosecond Laser assisted cataract surgery is one of the solutions with its ability to perform anterior capsulotomy, lens fragmentation, and to create self-sealing corneal incisions [155, 156]. The femtosecond laser (FSL) emits coherent optical pulses with a wavelength of 800 nm and duration on the order of 10 $^{-15}$ seconds. Due to its ability to alter delicate tissue in a precise and predictable way, it is used extensively in ophthalmology. Also, one of the major advantages is that it can cut tissue with almost no heat development. Today, there are many ongoing clinical studies utilizing the femtosecond lasers to perform several steps in cataract surgery such as incisions, capsulorhexis, and disassembly of the lens.

The femtosecond laser allows precision crafting of the lengths, angles, lanes, and shapes of clear corneal incisions to levels of consistency exceeding any manual technique [32]. Although

FLACS can be a promising surgical modality, there are questions of its widespread utility and accessibility [157]. The laser system such as LenSx (Alcon, Fort Worth, TX) produces a kHz pulse train of femtosecond pulses. In order to view the patients eye and to localize specific targets, an optical coherence tomography (OCT) imaging device and a video camera microscope are used. It is generally used for the creation of single plane and multi-plane incisions in the cornea, anterior capsulotomy and phacofragmentation. A beam of low energy pulses of infrared light is focused by the laser into the eye, leading to a micro-volume photodisruption of a tissue. After scanning the beam, numerous micro-disruptions are created in order to form an anterior capsulotomy incision as well as lens fragmentation incision, which are programmed depending on the location, shape, and size. [157-159]. Femtosecond laser assisted cataract surgery showed a lot of advantages in comparison to conventional cataract surgery. Some of them are less induced coma and astigmatism, manipulation, and phacoemulsification time [160]. A lot of arguments can be found in the literature regarding the increased risk of postoperative endophthalmitis following manually created clear corneal incision [161, 162]. In that matter, femtosecond laser assisted cataract surgery could be superior for it may allow for more square architecture, which has proven more resistant to leakage, added stability, and reproducibility at various intraocular pressures (IOPs) [163-165]. Femtosecond lasers also provide more accurate, safe, and adjustable cuts for limbal relaxing incisions, as well as predictable capsulorhexis [166]. Capsulorhexis performed with femtosecond laser has a higher degree of circularity, less risk for incomplete capsulorhexis-IOL overlap, better IOL centration [167, 168], and greater strength [168, 169]. It has been shown that the unpredictable diameter observed in manual capsulorhexis can have effects on IOL centration, with subsequent poor refractive outcomes, unpredictable anterior chamber depths, and increased rates of posterior capsular opacification [170-172].Some studies provided evidence of easier phacoemulsification performed with femtosecond laser [165, 173], reduced ultrasound energy for all grades of cataract [173, 174], and even more predictable IOL power calculations with laser assisted cataract surgery [175]. Taking into account that ultrasound phacoemulsification could damage the corneal tissue [176, 177], femtosecond laser assisted cataract surgery promises improved safety and lesser complications in that way also. On the other hand, patients with dementia, tremor, or with deep set orbits might not be good candidates for FLACS, as well as patients with poor dilated pupil, posterior synechiae, iris floppy syndrome, small eyelid fissure, and ocular motor paralysis [157].

Long-term clinical studies of the outcomes of the femtosecond laser assisted cataract surgery will provide evidence for the confirmation of its superiority over phacoemulsification.

11. Conclusion

The procedure of phacoemulsification revolutionized cataract surgery, especially since the introduction of sutureless clear corneal cataract incisions, which has led to reduced surgical time, lower induced astigmatism, faster postoperative and visual recovery, and less complications. Advances in technology and knowledge from the fields of optics and biomaterials have led to the development of minimally invasive procedures, as well as numerous various premium intraocular lenses that are designed to enable the best refractive outcomes with one goal: restoration of vision for distance and near and spectacles independence. The development of acrylic materials with a higher index of refraction and square edge designed intraocular lenses in order to prevent posterior capsular opacification led to patients having portions of their retina exposed to reflected light from the optic edge ending with dysphotopsia on the other hand. To achieve the best possible postoperative result, careful selection of patients, individual approach, and patient's education is mandatory.

In order to increase accuracy and precision in cataract surgery, together with patient demands for additional safety, femtosecond laser assisted cataract surgery is offered and being investigated as one of the possible solutions. As it appears safe and with many benefits in providing the best possible outcomes for cataract surgery, it stays on long-term clinical studies to provide evidence for the confirmation of its superiority over phacoemulsification.

Author details

Sanja Masnec * and Miro Kalauz

*Address all correspondence to: sanjamp@yahoo.com

Department of Ophthalmology, Zagreb University Hospital Centre, Zagreb, Croatia

References

[1] Kuszak JR, Deutsch TA, Brown HG. Anatomy of aged and senile cataractous lenses. In: Albert DM, Jakobiec FA, eds. Principles and Practice of Ophthalmology. Philadelphia: Saunders;1994: 564-75

[2] Lens and Cataract; American Academy of Ophthamology; Surgery for Cataract, 81-160

[3] Al Mahmood AM, Al-Swailem SA, Behrens A. Clear Corneal Incision in Cataract Surgery. Middle East Afr J Ophthalmol. 2014; Jan-Mar; 21(1): 25-31.doi: 10.4103/0974-9233.124084

[4] Fine IH. Clear corneal incisions. Int Ophthalmol Clin. 1994; 34: 59–72

[5] Girard LJ, Rodriguez J, Mailman ML. Reducing surgically induced astigmatism by using a scleral tunnel. Am J Ophthalmol. 1984; 97: 450–6

[6] Samuelson SW, Koch DD, Kuglen CC. Determination of maximal incision length for true small-incision surgery. Ophthalmic Surg. 1991; 22: 204–7

[7]   Ernest PH, Lavery KT, Kiessling LA. Relative strength of scleral corneal and clear corneal incisions constructed in cadaver eyes. J Cataract Refract Surg. 1994; 20 (6): 626–9

[8]   Ernest PH, Fenzl R, Lavery KT, Sensoli A. Relative stability of clear corneal incisions in a cadaver eye model. J Cataract Refract Surg. 1995; 21 (1): 39–42

[9]   Ernest P, Tipperman R, Eagle R. et al. Is there a difference in incision healing based on location?. J Cataract Refract Surg. 1998 ; 24 (4): 482–6

[10] Snell RS, Lemp MA. Clinical Anatomy of the Eye, Blackwell Science, Malden, MA, 2nd edition: 1998

[11] Ernest P, Hill W, Potvin R. Minimizing Surgically Induced Astigmatism at the Time of Cataract Surgery Using a Square Posterior Limbal Incision. J Ophthalmol. 2011; 24317.doi: 10.1155 2011/ 243170 Epub 2011 Nov 2

[12] ESCRS Endophthalmitis Study Group. Prophylaxis of postoperative endophthalmitis following cataract surgery: results of the ESCRS multicenter study and identification of risk factors. J ataract Refract Surg. 2007; 33 (6):978–88

[13] Cillino S, Morreale D, Mauceri A, Ajovalasit C, Ponte F. Temporal versus superior approach phacoemulsification: short-term postoperative astigmatism. J Cataract Refract Surg.1997; 23 (1997): 267-71

[14] Cravy TV. Routine use of a lateral approach to cataract extraction to achive rapid and sustained stabilisation of postoperative astigmatism. J Cataract Refract Surg. 1991; 17 (1991): 415-23

[15] Hayashi K, Nakao F, Hayashi F. Corneal topographic analysis of superolateral incision cataract surgery. Cataract Refract Surg. 1994; 20(1994): 392-9

[16] Simsek S, Yasar T, Demirok A. Effect of superior and temporal clear corneal incisions on astigmatism after sutureless phacoemulsification. J Cataract Refract Surg; 24(1998): 515-18

[17] Mendivil A. Comparative study of astigmatism through superior and lateral small incisions. Eur J Ophthalmol. 1996; 6 (1996): 389-92

[18] Rainer G, Menapace R, Vass C. Corneal shape changes after temporal and superolateral 3.0 mm clear corneal incisions. J Cataract Refract Surg. 1999; 25 (1999): 1121-26

[19] Wirbelauer C, Anders N, Pham DT, Wollensak J. Effect of incision location on preoperative oblique astigmatism after scleral tunnel incision. Cataract Refract Surg.1997; 23((1997): 365-71

[20] Ermis SS, Inan UU, Ozturk F. J Cataract Refract Surg. 2004; 30 (2004):1316-19

[21] Jacobs BJ, Gaynes BI, Deutch TA. Refractive astigmatism after oblique clear corneal phacoemulsification cataract incision. J Cataract Refract Surg. 1999; 25 (1999):949-52

[22] Brian J, Jacobs BS, Bruce I, Gaynes OD, Phar MD, Thomas A, Deutch MD. J Cataract Refractive Surg. 27 (2001):1176-9

[23] Masnec-Paškvalin S, Čima I, Iveković R, Matejčić A, Novak-Lauš K, Mandić Z. Comparison of Preoperative and Postoperative Astigmatism after Superotemporal or Superonasal Clear Corneal Incision in Phacoemulsiphication. Coll Antropol. 2007; 31(2007):199-202

[24] Azar DT, Stark WJ, Dodick J, Khoury JM., Vitale S, Enger C, Reed C. Prospective, randomized vector analysis of astigmatism after three-, one-, and no-suture phacoemulsification. J Cataract Refract Surg. 1997;23 (1997):1164-73

[25] Roman SJ, Auclin FX, Chong-Sit DA, Ullern MM. Surgically induced astigmatism with superior and temporal incisions in cases of with-the-rule preoperative astigmatism. J Cataract Refract Surg. 1998; 24 (1998):1636-41

[26] Masket S, Wang L, Belani S. Induced astigmatism with 2.2- and 3.0-mm coaxial phacoemulsification incisions. J Cataract Refract Surg. 2009; 25 (1): 21–24

[27] Hayashi K, Yoshida M, Hayashi H. Corneal shape changes after 2.0-mm or 3.0-mm clear corneal versus scleral tunnel incision cataract surgery. Ophthalmology.2010; 117 (7): 1313–23

[28] Pfleger T, Skorpik C, Menapace R, Scholz U, Weghaupt H, Zehetmayer M. Long-term course of induced astigmatism after clear corneal incision cataract surgery.JCataract Refract Surg. 1996; 22 (1): 72–7

[29] Buzard KA, Febbraro JL. Transconjunctival corneoscleral tunnel "blue line" cataract incision. J Cataract Refract Surg. 2000; 26:242–9

[30] Hurvitz LM. Late clear corneal wound failure after trivial trauma. J Cataract Refract Surg. 1999; 25: 283–4

[31] Fine IH, Fichman RA, Grabow HB. Clear-corneal cataract surgery and topical anesthesia. Slack Inc. 1993:29–62

[32] Dewey S, Beiko G, Braga-Mele R, Nixon DR, Raviv T, Rosenthal K. Microincisions in cataract surgery. J Cataract Refract Surg 2014; 40:1549-57

[33] Soscia W, Howard JG, Olson RJ. Microphacoemulsification with WhiteStar; a wound-temperature study. J Cataract Refract Surg. 2002; 28: 1044–6

[34] Payne M, Waite A, Olson RJ. Thermal inertia associated with ultrapulse technology in phacoemulsification. J Cataract Refract Surg. 2006; 32: 1032–4

[35] Han YK, Miller KM. Heat production: longitudinal versus torsional phacoemulsification. J Cataract Refract Surg. 2009; 35: 1799–805

[36] Devgan U. Phaco Fundamentals for the Beginning Phaco Surgeon. Bausch and Lomb Ophthalmology World Report Series, 2009: 1-54

[37] Georgescu D, Kuo AF, et al. A fluidics comparison of Alcon Infinity, Bausch and Lomb Stellaris, and Advanced Medical Optics Signature phacoemulsification machines. Am J Ophthalmol 2008; 145 (6): 1014-7

[38] Devgan U. Cataract surgery, Examining the differences between peristaltic and venturi pumps, OSN SuperSite, 2006

[39] Iancu R, Corbu C. Premium Intraocular Lenses Use in Patients with Cataract and Concurrent Glaucoma: a review. Maedica (Buchar). 2013; 8(3): 290-6

[40] Baumeister M, Kohnen T. Akkommodation und Presbyopie. Teil 1: Physiologie der Akkommodation und Entwicklung der Presbyopie (Accommodation and presbyopia. Part 1: physiology of accommodation and development of presbyopia). Ophthalmologe. 2008; 105: 597–608

[41] Keates RH, Pearce JL, Schneider RT. Clinical results of the multifocal lens. J Cataract Refract Surg. 1987;13:557–60

[42] Hansen TE, Corydon L, Krag S, et al. New multifocal intraocular lens design. J Cataract Refract Surg. 1990;16: 38–41

[43] Fresnel A. Imprimerie Royale Paris; France: 1822. Juillet. Memoire Sur un Nouveau Systeme d'Eclairage des Phares

[44] Chian PJ, Chan JH, Haider SI, et al. Multifocal IOLs Produce Similar Patient Satisfaction Levels. J Cataract Refract Surg. 2007; 33: 2057–61

[45] Packer M, Chu YR, Waltz KL, et al. Evaluation of the aspheric Tecnis multifocal intraocular lens: one-year results from the first cohort of the Food and Drug Administration clinical trial. Am J Ophthalmol. 2010; 149: 577–84

[46] Cillino S, Casuccio A, Di Pace F, et al. One-year outcomes with new-generation multifocal intraocular lenses. Ophthalmology. 2008; 115: 1508–16

[47] Gierek-Ciaciura S, Cwalina L, Bednarski L, et al. A comparative clinical study of the visual results between three types of multifocal lenses. Graefes Arch Clin Exp Ophthalmol. 2010; 248:133–40

[48] Alfonso JF, Fernandez -Vega L, Puchades C, et al. Intermediate visual function with different multifocal intraocularlens models. J Cataract Refract Surg. 2010; 36: 733–9

[49] de Vries NF, Nuijts RM. Multifocal intraocular lenses in cataract surgery: Literature review of benefits and side effects. J Cataract Refract Surg. 2013; 39: 268–78

[50] Montes-Mico R, Ferrer-Blasco T, Cervino A. Analysis of the possible benefits of aspheric intraocular lenses. J Cataract Refract Surg. 2009; 35: 172–181

[51] de Vries NF, Webers CA, Verbakel F, et al. Visual outcome and patient satisfaction after multifocal intraocular lens implantation: Aspheric versus spherical design. J Cataract Refract Surg. 2010; 36:1897–904

[52] Harman FE, Maling S, Kampougeris G, Langan L, Khan I, Lee N, Bloom PA. Comparing the 1CU accommodative, multifocal, and monofocal intraocular lenses; a randomized trial. Ophthalmology. 2008; 115: 993–1001

[53] Zhao G, Zhang J, Zhou Y, Hu L, Che C, Jiang N. Visual function after monocular implantation of apodized diffractive multifocal or single-piece monofocal intraocular lens; randomized prospective comparison. J Cataract Refract Surg. 2010; 36: 282–285

[54] Nijkamp MD, Dolders MGT, de Brabander J, van den Borne B, Hendrikse F, Nuijts RMMA. Effectiveness of multifocal intraocular lenses to correct presbyopia after cataract surgery; a randomized controlled trial. Ophthalmology. 2004; 111: 1832–9

[55] Sen HN, Sarikkola AU, Uusitalo RJ, Laatikainen L. Quality of vision after AMO Array multifocal intraocular lens implantation. J Cataract Refract Surg. 2004; 30: 2483–93

[56] Zeng M, Liu Y, Liu X, Yuan Z, Luo L, Xia Y, Zeng Y. Aberration and contrast sensitivity comparison of aspherical and monofocal and multifocal intraocular lens eyes. Clin Exp Ophthalmol. 2007; 35: 355–60

[57] Leyland M, Zinicola E. Multifocal versus monofocal intraocular lenses in cataract surgery; a systematic review. Ophthalmology. 2003; 110: 1789–98

[58] Leyland M, Pringle E. Multifocal versus monofocal intraocular lenses after cataract extraction. Cochrane Database Syst Rev. 2006; Oct 18 (4); CD003169

[59] Woodward MA, Randleman JB, Stulting RD. Dissatisfaction after multifocal intraocular lens implantation. J Cataract Refract Surg. 2009; 35: 992–997

[60] de Vries NE, Webers CAB, Touwslager WRH, Bauer NJC, de Brabander J, Berendschot TT, Nuijts RMMA. Dissatisfaction after implantation of multifocal intraocular lenses. J Cataract Refract Surg. 2011; 37: 859–65

[61] Chiam PJT, Chan JH, Aggarwal RK, Kasaby S. ReSTOR intraocular lens implantation in cataract surgery: quality of vision. J Cataract Refract Surg. 2006; 32: 1459–63

[62] Häring G, Dick HB, Krummenauer F, Weissmantel U, Kröncke W. Subjective photic phenomena with refractive multifocal and monofocal intraocular lenses; results of a multicenter questionnaire. J Cataract Refract Surg. 2001; 27: 245–9

[63] Mesci C, Erbil H, Özdöker L, Karakurt Y, Dolar Bilge A. Visual acuity and contrast sensitivity function after accommodative and multifocal intraocular lens implantation. Eur J Ophthalmol. 2010; 20: 90–100

[64] Mesci C, Erbil HH, Olgun, A, Aydin N, Candemir B, Akçakaya AA. Differences in contrast sensitivity between monofocal, multifocal and accommodating intraocular lenses: long-term results. Clin Exp Ophthalmol. 2010; 38: 768–77

[65] Ortiz D, Alió JL, Bernabéu G, Pongo V. Optical performance of monofocal and multifocal intraocular lenses in the human eye. J Cataract Refract Surg. 2008; 34: 755–62

[66] Pepose JS, Qazi MA, Davies J, Doane JF, Loden JC, Sivalingham V, Mahmoud AM. Visual performance of patients with bilateral vs combination Crystalens, ReZoom, and ReSTOR intraocular lens implants. Am J Ophthalmol. 2007; 144: 347–57

[67] Kohnen T, Nuijts R, Levy P, Haefliger E, Alfonso JF. Visual function after bilateral implantation of apodized diffractive aspheric multifocal intraocular lenses with a +3.0 D addition. J Cataract Refract Surg. 2009; 35: 2062–9

[68] Gatinel D, Pagnoulle C, Houbrechts Y, Gobin L. Design and qualification of a diffractive trifocal optical profile for intraocular lenses. J Cataract Refract Surg. 2011; 37: 2060–7

[69] Pepose JS. Maximizing satisfaction with presbyopia-correcting intraocular lenses: the missing links. Am J Ophthalmol. 2008; 146: 641–8

[70] Lichtinger A, Rootman DS. Intraocular lenses for presbyopia correction: past, present, and future. Curr Opin Ophthalmol. 2012; 23: 40–6

[71] Doane John F, Jacksob RT. Accommodaive intraocular lenses: considerations on use, function and design. Curr Opin Ophthalmol. 2007;18: 318-24

[72] Shepard A, Wolffsohn JS. Accommodating intraocular lenses: past, present, future. Ophthalmology international. 2011; 6:45–52

[73] Klaproth OK, Titke C, Baumeister M, et al. Accommodative intraocular lenses-principles of clinical evaluation and current results. Klinische Monatsblätter für Augenheilkunde. 2011; 228: 666–75

[74] Nishi Y, Mireskandari K, Khaw P, Findl O. Lens refilling to restore accommodation. J Cataract Refract Surg. 2009; 35: 374–82

[75] Menapace R, Findl O, Kriechbaum K, Leydolt-Koeppl C. Accommodating intraocular lenses: a critical review of present and future concepts. Graefes Arch Clin Exp Ophthalmol. 2007; 245: 473–89

[76] Marchini G, Pedrotti E, Modesti M, Visentin S, Tosi R. Anterior segment changes during accommodation in eyes with a monofocal intraocular lens: high-frequency ultrasound study. J Cataract Refract Surg. 2008; 34: 949–56

[77] Koeppl C, Findl O, Kriechbaum K, Sacu C, Drexler W. Change in IOL position and capsular bag size with an angulated intraocular lens early after cataract surgery. J Cataract Refract Surg. 2005; 31: 348–53

[78] Koeppl C, Findl O, Menapace R, Kriechbaum K, Wirtitsch M, Buehl W, Sacu S, Drexler W. Pilocarpine-induced shift of an accommodating intraocular lens: AT-45 Crystalens. J Cataract Refract Surg. 2005; 31: 1290–7

[79] Findl O, Leydolt C. Meta-analysis of accommodating intraocular lenses. J Cataract Refract Surg. 2007; 33: 522–7

[80] Hoffer KJ. Biometry of 7, 500 cataractous eyes. Am J Ophthalmol. 1980; 90: 360–8

[81] Ferrer-Blasco T, Montés-Micó R, Peixoto-de-Matos SC, González-Méijome JM, Cerviño A. Prevalence of corneal astigmatism before cataract surgery. J Cataract Refract Surg. 2009; 35: 70–5

[82] Hoffmann PC, Hütz WW. Analysis of biometry and prevalence data for corneal astigmatism in 23, 239 eyes. J Cataract Refract Surg. 2010; 36: 1479–85

[83] Visser N, Bauer NJC, Nuijts MR, Toric intraocular lenses: Historical overview, patient selection, IOL calculation, surgical techniques, clinical outcomes, and complications, J Cataract Refract Surg. 2013;39:624-37

[84] Buckhurst PJ, Wolffsohn JS, Davies LN, Naroo SA. Surgical correction of astigmatism during cataract surgery. Clin Exp Optom 2010; 93:409-18.

[85] Amesbury EC, Miller KM. Correction of astigmatism at thr time of cataract surgery. Curr Opin Ophthalmol 2009; 20:19-24

[86] Grabow HB. Early results with foldable toric IOL implantation. Eur J Implant Refract Surg. 1994; 6: 177–8

[87] Grabow HB. Toric intraocular lens report. Ann Ophthalmol Glaucoma. 1997; 29: 161–3

[88] Sun XY, Vicary D, Montgomery P, Griffiths M. Toric intraocular lenses for correcting astigmatism in 130 eyes. Ophthalmology. 2000; 107: 1776–81 (discussion by RM Kershner, 1781–2)

[89] Ruhswurm I, Scholz U, Zehetmayer M, Hanselmayer G, Vass C, Skorpik C. Astigmatism correction with a foldable toric intraocular lens in cataract patients. J Cataract Refract Surg. 2000; 26: 1022–7

[90] Linnola RJ, Werner L, Pandey SK, Escobar-Gomez M, Znoiko SL, Apple DJ. Adhesion of fibronectin, vitronectin, laminin, and collagen type IV to intraocular lens materials in pseudophakic human autopsy eyes. Part 1: histological sections. J Cataract Refract Surg. 2000; 26: 1792–806

[91] Lombardo M, Carbone G, Lombardo G, De Santo MP, Barberi R. Analysis of intraocular lens surface adhesiveness by atomic force microscopy. J Cataract Refract Surg. 2009; 35: 1266–72

[92] Oshika T, Nagata T, Ishii Y. Adhesion of lens capsule to intraocular lenses of polymethylmethacrylate, silicone, and acrylic foldable materials: an experimental study. Br J Ophthalmol. 1998; 82: 549–53

[93] Patel CK, Ormonde S, Rosen PH, Bron AJ. Postoperative intraocular lens rotation: a randomized comparison of plate and loop haptic implants. Ophthalmology. 1999; 106: 2190–5 (discussion by DJ Apple, 2196)

[94] Chang DF. Early rotational stability of the longer Staar toric intraocular lens; fifty consecutive cases. J Cataract Refract Surg. 2003; 29: 935–40

[95] Shah GD, Praveen MR, Vasavada AR, Vasavada VA, Rampal G, Shastry LR. Rotational stability of a toric intraocular lens: influence of axial length and alignment in the capsular bag. J Cataract Refract Surg. 2012; 38: 54–9

[96] Prinz A, Neumayer T, Buehl W, Vock L, Menapace R, Findl O, Georgopoulos M. Rotational stability and posterior capsule opacification of a plate-haptic and an open-loop-haptic intraocular lens. J Cataract Refract Surg. 2011; 37: 251–7

[97] Visser N, Gast STJM, Bauer NJ, Nuijts RMM. Cataract surgery with toric intraocular lens implantation in keratoconus: a case report. Cornea. 2011; 30: 720–3

[98] Luck J. Customized ultra-high-power toric intraocular lens implantation for pellucid marginal degeneration and cataract. J Cataract Refract Surg. 2010; 36: 1235–8

[99] Kersey JP, O'Donnell A, Illingworth CD. Cataract surgery with toric intraocular lenses can optimize uncorrected postoperative visual acuity in patients with marked corneal astigmatism. Cornea. 2007; 26: 133–5

[100] Stewart, CM, McAlister JC. Comparison of grafted and non-grafted patients with corneal astigmatism undergoing cataract extraction with a toric intraocular lens implant. Clin Exp Ophthalmol. 2010; 38: 747–57

[101] Hayashi K, Manabe SI, Yoshida M, Hayashi H. Effect of astigmatism on visual acuity in eyes with a diffractive multifocal intraocular lens. J Cataract Refract Surg. 2010; 36: 1323–9

[102] Findl O, Buehl W, Bauer P, Sycha T. Interventions for preventing posterior capsule opacification. Cochrane Database System Rev 2010; Issue 2, Art. No. CD003738. DOI: 10.1002/14651858.CD003738.pub3.

[103] Buehl W, Findl O. Effect of intraocular lens design on posterior capsule opacification. J Cataract Refract Surg.2008; 34:1976–85

[104] Nishi O, Nishi K, Mano C, Ichihara M, Honda T. The inhibition of lens epithelial cell migration by a discontinuous capsular bend created by a band-shaped circular loop or a capsule-bending ring. Ophthalmic Surg Lasers. 1998;29:119–125

[105] Buehl W, Findl O, Menapace R, Rainer G, Sacu S, Kiss B, et al. Effect of an acrylic intraocular lens with a sharp posterior optic edge on posterior capsule opacification. J Cataract Refract Surg. 2002 ;28:1105–11

[106] Buehl W, Findl O, Menapace R, Sacu S, Kriechbaum K, Koeppl C, et al. Long-term effect of optic edge design in an acrylic intraocular lens on posterior capsule opacification. J Cataract Refract Surg. 2005; 31: 954–61

[107] Peng Q, Visessook N, Apple DJ, Pandey SK, Werner L, Escobar-Gomez M, et al. Surgical prevention of posterior capsule opacification. Part 3: intraocular lens optic barrier effect as a second line of defense. J Cataract Refract Surg.2000; 26: 198–213

[108] Kohnen T, Fabian E, Gerl R, Hunold W, Hütz W, Strobel J, et al. Optic edge design as long-term factor for posterior capsular opacification rates. Ophthalmology. 2008;115: 1308–14

[109] Kugelberg M, Wejde G, Jayaram H, Zetterström C. Posterior capsule opacification after implantation of a hydrophilic or a hydrophobic acrylic intraocular lens; one-year follow-up. J Cataract Refract Surg. 2006; 32: 1627–31

[110] Johansson B. Clinical consequences of acrylic intraocular lens material and design: Nd:YAG-laser capsulotomy rates in 3 x 300 eyes 5 years after phacoemulsification. Br J Ophthalmol. 2010; 94: 450–5

[111] Apple DJ, Ram J, Foster A, Peng Q. Posterior capsule opacification (secondary cataract). Surv Ophthalmol. 2000;45(suppl 1):S100–S130

[112] Vasavada AR, Raj SM, Johar K, Nanavaty MA. Effect of hydrodissection alone and hydrodissection combined with rotation on lens epithelial cells; surgical approach for the prevention of posterior capsule opacification. J Cataract Refract Surg.2006; 32: 145–150

[113] Kugelberg M, Wejde G, Jayaram H, Zetterström C. Two-year follow-up of posterior capsule opacification after implantation of a hydrophilic or hydrophobic acrylic intraocular lens. Acta Ophthalmol (Oxf). 2008; 86: 533–6

[114] Vasavada AR, Shah A, Raj SM, Praveen MR, Shah GD. Prospective evaluation of posterior capsule opacification in myopic eyes 4 years after implantation of a single-piece acrylic IOL. J Cataract Refract Surg. 2009; 35: 1532–9

[115] Khandwala MA, Marjanovic B, Kotagiri AK, Teimory M. Rate of posterior capsule opacification in eyes with the Akreos intraocular lens. J Cataract Refract Surg. 2007; 33:1409–13

[116] Heatley CJ, Spalton DJ, Kumar A, Jose R, Boyce J, Bender LE. Comparison of posterior capsule opacification rates between hydrophilic and hydrophobic single-piece acrylic intraocular lenses. J Cataract Refract Surg. 2005; 31: 718–24

[117] Hayashi K, Hayashi H. Posterior capsule opacification after implantation of a hydrogel intraocular lens. Br J Ophthalmol.2004; 88: 182–5

[118] Halpern MT, Covert D, Battista C, et al. Relationship of AcrySof acrylic and PhacoFlex silicone intraocular lenses to visual acuity and posterior capsule opacification. J Cataract Refract Surg. 2002; 28: 662–9

[119] Nishi O, Nishi K, Wickström K. Preventing lens epithelial cell migration using intraocular lenses with sharp rectangular edges. J Cataract Refract Surg. 2000; 26: 1543–9

[120] Nishi O, Yamamoto N, Nishi K, Nishi Y. Contact inhibition of migrating lens epithelial cells at the capsular bend created by a sharp-edged intraocular lens after cataract surgery. J Cataract Refract Surg. 2007; 33: 1065–70

[121] Werner L, Mamalis N, Pandey SK, Izak AM, Nilson CD, Davis BL, et al. Posterior capsule opacification in rabbit eyes implanted with hydrophilic acrylic intraocular lenses with enhanced square edge. J Cataract Refract Surg. 2004; 30: 2403–9

[122] Li N, Chen X, Zhang J, Zhou Y, Yao X, Du L, et al. Effect of AcrySof versus silicone or polymethyl methacrylate intraocular lens on posterior capsule opacification. Ophthalmology. 2008; 115(5) :830–8

[123] Farbowit MA, Zabriskie NA, Crandall AS, Olson RJ, Miller KM. Visual complaints associated with the AcrySof acrylic intraocular lens(1). J Cataract Refract Surg. 2000; 26:1339-45

[124] Holladay JT, Lang A, Portney V. Analysis of edge glare phenomena in intraocular lens edge designs. J Cataract Refract Surg. 1999; 25: 748-52

[125] Holladay JT, Zhao H, Reisin CR. Negative dysphotopsia: the enigmatic penumbra. J Cataract Refract Surg. 2012; 38: 1251-65

[126] Davison JA. Positive and negative dysphotopsia in patients with acrylic intraocular lenses.J Cataract Refract Surg. 2000; 26:1346-56

[127] Radford SW, Carlsson AM, Barrett GD. Comparison of pseudophakic dysphotopsia with Akreos Adapt and SN60-AT intraocular lenses. J Cataract Refract Surg. 2007; 33: 88-93

[128] Narvaez J, Banning CS, Stulting RD. Negative dysphotopsia associated with implantation of the Z9000 intraocular lens.J Cataract Refract Surg. 2005; 31: 846-7

[129] Erie JC, Bandhauer MH, McLaren JW. Analysis of postoperative glare and intraocular lens design. J Cataract Refract Surg. 2001; 27: 614- 21

[130] Erie JC, Bandhauer MH. Intraocular lens surfaces and their relationship to postoperative glare. J Cataract Refract Surg. 2003; 29: 336-41

[131] Vamosi P, Csakany B, Nemeth J. Intraocular lens exchange in patients with negative dysphotopsia symptoms.J Cataract Refract Surg. 2010; 36: 418- 24

[132] Osher RH. Negative dysphotopsia: long-term study and possible explanation for transient symptoms. J Cataract Refract Surg. 2008; 34: 1699- 707

[133] Gossala S. Optical phenomena causing negative dysphotopsia. Cataract Refract Surg. 2010; 36: 1620-1

[134] Masket S, Fram NR. Pseudophakic negative dysphotopsia: Surgical management and new theory of etiology. J Cataract Refract Surg. 2011; 37: 1199- 207

[135] Izak AM, Werner L, Pandey SK. Single-piece hydrophobic acrylic intraocular lens explanted within the capsular bag: case report with clinicopathological correlation. Cataract Refract Surg. 2004; 30: 1356- 61

[136] Weinstein A. Surgical experience with pseudophakic negative dysphotopsia. J Cataract Refract Surg. 2012; 38: 561

[137] Jin Y, Zabriskie N, Olson RJ. Dysphotopsia outcomes analysis of two truncated acrylic 6.0-mm intraocular optic lenses. Ophthalmol. 2009; 223: 47- 51

[138] Sambhu S, Shanmuganathan VA, Charles SJ. The effect of lens design on dysphotopsia in different acrylic IOLs. Eye. 2005; 19: 567-70

[139] Kinard K, Jarstad A, Olson RJ. Correlation of visual quality with satisfaction and function in a normal cohort of pseudophakic. J Cataract Refract Surg. 2013; 39: 590 -7

[140] Holladay JT. Reply: Etiology of negative dysphotopsia. J Cataract Refract Surg. 2013; 39: 486- e1- 4

[141] Bournas B, Drazinos S, Kanellas D, Arvanitis M, Vaikoussis E. Dysphotopsia after cataract surgery: comparison of four different intraocular lenses. Ophthalmol. 2007; 221: 378 - 83

[142] Miyoshi T. J Cataract Refract Surg. 2006 ; 32 : 912

[143] Stulting D. Consultation section. Cataract surgical problem. J Cataract Refract Surg. 2005; 31: 651- 60

[144] Arnold PN. Photic phenomena after phacoemulsification and posterior chamber lens implantation of various optic sizes. J Cataract Refract Surg. 1994; 20: 446 - 50

[145] Tratler WB. J Cataract Refract Surg. 2011; 37: 1199

[146] Folden DV. Neodymium:YAG laser anterior capsulectomy: surgical option in the management of negative dysphotopsia.J Cataract Refract Surg. 2013; 39: 1110-5

[147] Cooke DL, Kasko S, Platt LO. Resolution of negative dysphotopsia after laser anterior capsulotomy. J Cataract Refract Surg. 2013; 39: 1107- 9

[148] Davison JA. Clinical performance of Alcon SA30AL and SA60AT single-piece acrylic intraocular lenses. J Cataract Refract Surg. 2002; 28: 1112- 23

[149] Davison JA. J Cataract Refract Surg. 2005; 31: 657

[150] Tester R, Pace NL, Samore M, Olson RJ. Dysphotopsia in phakic and pseudophakic patients: incidence and relation to intraocular lens type(2). J Cataract Refract Surg. 2000; 26: 810-5

[151] Hong X, Liu Y, Karakelle M, Masket S, Fram NR. Ray-tracing optical modeling of negative dysphotopsia. J Biomed Opt. 2011; 16: 125001

[152] Walkow T, Anders N, Pham DT, Wollensak J. Causes of severe decentration and subluxation of intraocular lenses. Graefes Arch Clin Exp Ophthalmol. 1998; 236: 9–12

[153] Cekic O, Batman C. The relationship between capsulorhexis size and anterior chamber depth relation. Ophthalmic Surg Lasers. 1999; 30:185–190

[154] Wolffsohn JS, Buckhurst PJ. Objective analysis of toric intraocular lens rotation and centration. J Cataract Refract Surg. 2010; 36: 778–82

[155] Nagy ZZ. 1-year clinical experience with a new femtosecond laser for refractive cataract surgery; Paper presented at: Annual Meeting of the American Academy of Ophthalmology; 2009: San Francisco, CA

[156] Nagy ZZ. Intraocular femtosecond laser applications in cataract surgery. Cataract & Refractive Surgery Today. 2009 Sep; 79–82

[157] Chen Ming, A review of femtosecond laser assisted cataract surgery for Hawaii, Hawaii J Med Public Health. May 2013; 72(5): 152 – 5

[158] Krasnov MM. Laser-phakopuncture in the treatment of soft cataracts. Br J Ophthalmol. 1975; 59:96–8

[159] Peyman GA, Katoh N. Effects of an erbium: YAG laser on ocular structures. Int Ophthalmol. 1987; 10: 245–53

[160] Slade SG. Illinois, USA: 2010. Oct 15–16, First 50 accommodating IOLs with an image-guided femtosecond laser in cataract surgery. Program and Abstracts of the Annual Meeting of ISRS

[161] Taban M, Behrens A, Newcomb RL, Nobe MY, Saedi G, Sweet PM, et al. Acute endophthalmitis following cataract surgery: A systematic review of the literature. Arch Ophthalmol. 2005; 123: 613–20

[162] Xia Y, Liu X, Luo L, Zeng Y, Cai X, Zeng M, et al. Early changes in clear cornea incision after phacoemulsification: An anterior segment optical coherence tomography study. Acta Ophthalmol. 2009; 87: 764–8

[163] Ernest PH, Kiessling LA, Lavery KT. Relative strength of cataract incisions in cadaver eyes. J Cataract Refract Surg. 1991; 17(Suppl): 668–71

[164] Masket S, Sarayba M, Ignacio T, Fram N. Femtosecond laser-assisted cataract incisions: Architectural stability and reproducibility. J Cataract Refract Surg. 2010; 36: 1048–9

[165] Palanker DV, Blumenkranz MS, Andersen D, Wiltberger M, Marcellino G, Gooding P, et al. Femtosecond laser-assisted cataract surgery with integrated optical coherence tomography. Sci Transl Med. 2010; 2:58ra85

[166] Trivedi RH, Wilson ME, Jr, Bartholomew LR. Extensibility and scanning electron microscopy evaluation of 5 pediatric anterior capsulotomy techniques in a porcine model. J Cataract Refract Surg. 2006; 32: 1206–13

[167] Kránitz K, Takacs A, Mihaltz K, Kovacs I, Knorz MC, Nagy ZZ. Femtosecond laser capsulotomy and manual continuous curvilinear capsulorhexis parameters and their effects on intraocular lens centration. J Refract Surg. 2011:1–6

[168] Nagy Z, Takacs A, Filkorn T, Sarayba M. Initial clinical evaluation of an intraocular femtosecond laser in cataract surgery. J Refract Surg. 2009; 25:1053–60

[169] Friedman NJ, Palanker DV, Schuele G, Andersen D, Marcellino G, Seibel BS, et al. Femtosecond laser capsulotomy. J Cataract Refract Surg. 2011; 37:1189–98

[170] Dick HB, Pena-Aceves A, Manns M, Krummenauer F. New technology for sizing the continuous curvilinear capsulorhexis: Prospective trial. J Cataract Refract Surg. 2008; 34: 1136–44

[171] Norrby S. Sources of error in intraocular lens power calculation. J Cataract Refract Surg. 2008; 34: 368–76

[172] Hollick EJ, Spalton DJ, Meacock WR. The effect of capsulorhexis size on posterior capsular opacification: One-year results of a randomized prospective trial. Am J Ophthalmol. 1999; 128: 271–9

[173] Koch D, Batlle J, Feliz R, Friedman N, Seibel B. Paris, France: 2010. Sep 4–10, the use of OCT- guided femtosecond laser to facilitate cataract nuclear disassembly and aspiration [abstract] Program and Abstracts of XXVIII Congress of the ESCRS

[174] Fishkind W, Uy H, Tackman R, Kuri J. Boston, MA: 2010. Apr 9–14, Alternative fragmentation patterns in femtosecond laser cataract surgery [abstract] Program and Abstracts of American Society of Cataract and Refractive Surgeons Symposium on Cataract, IOL and Refractive Surgery

[175] Filkorn T, Kovacs I, Takacs A, et al. Comparison of IOL power calculation and refractive outcome after laser refractive cataract surgery with a femtosecond laser versus conventional phacoemulsification. J Refract Surg. 2012; 28(8): 540–4

[176] Murano N, Ishizaki M, Sato S, Fukuda Y, Takahashi H. Corneal endothelial cell damage by free radicals associated with ultrasound oscillation. Arch Ophthalmol. 2008; 126: 816–21

[177] Shin YJ, Nishi Y, Engler C, Kang J, Hashmi S, Jun AS, et al. The effect of phacoemulsification energy on the redox state of cultured human corneal endothelial cells. Arch Ophthalmol. 2009; 127: 435–41

2

Diagnostic Procedures in Ophthalmology

Roy Schwartz and Zohar Habot-Wilner

Abstract

Determining the cause of intraocular inflammation has important implications both for the treatment and prognosis of uveitic diseases. This chapter describes ocular diagnostic procedures and their indications while mainly focusing on diagnostic vitrectomy. The chapter discusses the history of elective diagnostic procedures; main indications for invasive procedures in the diagnosis of uveitic disease; surgical principles and techniques for each of the diagnostic procedures; descriptions of the various laboratory techniques being used; and selected examples of conditions that may require the use of such techniques.

Keywords: Uveitis, diagnostic vitrectomy, tap

1. Introduction

The term uveitis refers to a large and varied group of disease entities, each with its own set of manifestations. While some may fit textbook characteristics, others may present in a way that baffles us as clinicians and leaves us with a wide differential diagnosis. Determining the cause of intraocular inflammation has important implications both for treatment and for prognosis of the disease. That is where the field of invasive diagnostic procedures comes into place. Through the use of different laboratory techniques, this diagnostic modality adds to the battery of other methods available to the clinician in order to reach the final diagnosis and provide proper management.

This chapter covers ocular diagnostic procedures, while focusing mainly on diagnostic vitrectomy.

2. History

The earliest attempts at elective pars plana vitreous surgery were directed toward cutting opaque vitreous. While still not used for the diagnosis of the etiology, papers as early as the 19th century report on the procedure in the context of ocular inflammation. Bull reported in 1890 on 17 cases in which a pars plana approach (first introduced by Von Graefe in 1863) involving a discission needle introduced through the pars plana was used to cut vitreous membranes resulting from inflammation or hemorrhage. [1]

The 1970s were a period of major advancement in the field of pars plana vitrectomy (PPV), with the introduction of advanced instrumentation, such as the vitreous-infusion-suction-cutter (VISC). Indications for diagnostic procedures and the diagnostic methods themselves were limited at that time. In a review paper from 1974, Michels et al. [1] described vitreous biopsy as a procedure that is rarely needed, with the most frequent indications being mycotic endophthalmitis and reticulum cell sarcoma. The diagnostic methods that were mentioned included only cytology and culture. Vitrectomy for endophthalmitis was also mentioned in this paper, and showed that performing the procedure for this entity was a novelty.

One of the first papers to describe diagnostic vitrectomy was published by Engel et al in 1981. [2] Findings resulting from early procedures in that era included ocular tumors such as reticulum cell sarcoma and leukemic infiltration, as well as infectious entities such as fungal endophthalmitis and acute retinal necrosis (ARN). The methods described there included cytology, histopathology, and ultrastructural studies, with "new" methods such as using a millipore filter and celloidin-bag cell-block techniques.

Since these early days, the field of diagnostic procedures has advanced rapidly. Methods including polymerase chain reaction (PCR), flow cytometry, and other advanced methods introduced in the general field of medicine have been adopted by ophthalmologists for use in ocular diagnostic procedures. With the introduction of these methods, the list of etiologies that can be recognized by invasive diagnostic techniques has also expanded, as will be described here.

3. Indications

Accurate diagnosis of the etiology behind intraocular inflammation is essential in order to provide the proper treatment and management and for prognostic reasons. While the general approach to uveitis patients includes history taking, review of systems, examination, and ancillary tests, at times none of these result in a conclusive diagnosis. In these atypical cases a diagnostic vitrectomy may lead to the correct diagnosis. An example for such an indication is primary intraocular lymphoma (PIOL), which requires a definitive tissue diagnosis to diagnose and commence treatment.[3]

Another indication for this procedure is failure of conventional therapy. While this might result from an intractable disease, it may also be the result of a misdiagnosis, requiring an invasive approach to reach the correct diagnosis.

A third indication is a sight-threatening disease, where the disease rapidity necessitates an invasive approach for diagnosis, and at times also for treatment. Examples for infectious entities that correspond to this description include infectious endophthalmitis [4] and ARN. [5]

4. Surgical principles and techniques

Prior to the procedures described henceforth, an informed consent should be obtained from the patient after discussing the potential for complications. Since modern diagnostic techniques may require special preparation (e.g. special stains or cultures) the laboratory or pathologist should be notified of the procedure and upcoming samples, and any requirements regarding the handling of the sample prior to delivery should be noted.

4.1. Anterior chamber tap

Unlike diagnostic vitrectomy, an anterior chamber tap may be done in an office setting and is less invasive. It is important to note that this procedure yields a smaller amount of fluid for analysis in comparison with diagnostic vitrectomy, and as such may be considered in cases in which a small sample may suffice for diagnosis.

The procedure is done under an aseptic technique. The area around the eye is cleaned with povidone-iodine and a local anesthetic is instilled into the eye. It may be done at the slit lamp or with the patient in a supine position by using binocular loupes. The eye is opened and fixated with a speculum. The conjunctival surface is washed with povidone-iodine solution. A 27-30-gauge needle on a tuberculin syringe is inserted to the anterior chamber using a limbal approach, and 200 to 250 μL of fluid can be obtained. At the end of the procedure, an antibiotic drop and povidone-iodine solution is instilled into the eye and a broad spectrum antibiotic drop is prescribed for several days. [6, 7]

Anterior chamber tap is a relatively safe procedure. Possible complications include trauma to the cornea, lens, and iris; hyphema; corneal abscess; and endophthalmitis. However these complications are rare. [7]

4.2. Vitreous aspiration needle tap

A vitreous specimen for analysis can be obtained by straight needle vitreous aspiration, or vitreous tap. This procedure has the advantages of being easier to perform, being less traumatic to the eye than diagnostic vitrectomy, and offering the ability to perform it in an office setting. Disadvantages of vitreous aspiration include: (1) the risk for retinal detachment from vitreoretinal traction during aspiration [8]; (2) a smaller amount of specimen in comparison to diagnostic vitrectomy as the procedure only yields about 300 μL of ocular fluid [9], which allows for fewer diagnostic tests and possibly a lower yield; (3) it is also not therapeutic, as a diagnostic vitrectomy could be, since it does not clear a large amount of vitreous (and thus does not allow for better diffusion of intraocular medications, [10] removal of pathogens or improved media clarity [11, 12]).

The procedure is done under an aseptic technique. The area around the eye is cleaned with povidone-iodine and a local anesthetic is instilled into the eye. The eye is opened and fixated with a speculum and the conjunctival surface is washed with povidone-iodine solution. A large-caliber needle is usually needed, such as a 21-gauge hollow needle, mounted on a 1 ml syringe as an aspirating device, which permits better control during the procedure. The needle is directed posteriorly in the direction of the optic nerve head and vitreous humor is obtained. At the end of the procedure an antibiotic drop and povidone-iodine solution is instilled into the eye, and a broad spectrum antibiotic drop is prescribed for several days. [9]

4.3. Diagnostic vitrectomy

The aim of vitrectomy is to try to obtain the maximum possible amount of tissue from which a diagnosis can be made. A small sample volume may reduce the diagnostic yield. A variety of techniques involving the use of 20, 23, and 25 G PPV have been described in the literature. [13-19] An undiluted vitreous sample is obtained using a 3 or 5 mL syringe attached to the vitreous cutter. When the vitrector is cutting the vitreous, the assistant manually aspirates it until the eye softens, and the infusion is turned on. This provides between 1-2 mL of undiluted vitreous. Some authors propose using continuous infusion of air or perfluorocarbon liquid to substitute the vitreous removed from the eyeball which allows obtaining a larger amount of vitreous. [20, 21]

Following collection of undiluted specimen, fluid infusion is initiated and a second syringe is placed on the vitreous cutter to collect 3-10 mL of a diluted vitreous sample. [11, 15, 18] The surgeon may then proceed with core vitrectomy, induction of a posterior vitreous detachment, and peripheral vitrectomy using a standard approach if necessary. [16, 19, 21] Meticulous peripheral vitrectomy in the presence of significant media opacity, as may occur in many uveitis patients, is accompanied by potential complications and should generally be avoided. [21]

Complications

Diagnostic vitrectomy carries the possibility of complications encountered in vitrectomy for other indications, with some added due to the nature of the underlying etiology.

Cataract formation is a common complication after vitrectomy procedures reported to range from 12.5%-80% in 20-gauge PPV and 22.7%-79.3% in small gauge PPV. [22] The rate of cataract progression is higher in individuals older than 50 years. [23]

Retinal detachment is a possible complication of any PPV. In the setting of diagnostic vitrectomy, this complication may be related to the underlying etiology. For example, in cases of viral or fungal endophthalmitis it may already appear at the time of surgery, complicating the diagnostic procedure. [24]

Retinal detachment may also occur as a result of surgery. Iatrogenic retinal tears at the time of surgery may lead to retinal detachment. [25] This complication is especially true in ARN, where necrosis of the retina leads to its atrophy and subsequent retinal break formation. [26] It also may occur due to the development of new retinal breaks postoperatively.

Other, rarer complications of PPV include open-angle glaucoma, [27] retinal and vitreous incarceration, endophthalmitis, and vitreous hemorrhage. [28]

4.4. Chorioretinal biopsy

Chorioretinal biopsy should only be considered when the inflammatory process is localized primarily in the sensory retina, retinal pigment epithelium, or choroid and when in a previous workup neither aqueous nor vitreous samples provided the diagnostic answer. The main indication is diagnosis of a suspected intraocular lymphoma.

It is important to remember that this procedure involves a greater risk, including subretinal hemorrhage, vitreous hemorrhage, and retinal detachment, [29, 30] and should therefore only be used as a last resort.

The procedure may be done using 20 or 23 G 3-port PPV. Prior to the biopsy, undiluted and diluted vitreous samples are collected as described previously. The vitreous is separated over the biopsy site and intraocular diathermy is used to delineate the biopsy site and the border between the lesion and normal retina. A sample size of 1 x 1 mm or 2 x 2 mm is excised using vertical scissors or a diamond blade, while elevating the intraocular pressure temporarily to 70-90 mm Hg to prevent bleeding. The tissue is then grasped using intraocular forceps and removed through the sclerotomy site. Endolaser is applied around the biopsy site and the procedure is ended with long-acting gas or silicone tamponade. [21]

5. Diagnostic testing of vitreous specimens

With the advent of new laboratory techniques, a myriad of options are available for the clinician in the quest for obtaining a correct diagnosis of an unknown inflammatory, infectious, or neoplastic entity.

Of course not all tests should be performed in all cases, and tests should be chosen according to the suspected diagnosis.

5.1. Histopathologic evaluation

A sample is sent to a pathologist following the diagnostic procedure and is immediately processed. The specimen is generally divided into three portions: one third is fixed for routine histopathological evaluation, including light and electron microscopic examination. Another one third is frozen in optimal cutting temperature (OCT) embedding compound for immu-nopathology (phenotyping of cells by their surface markers) and molecular characterization. The last third portion is sent for culture of microorganisms. If the specimen is not adequate for all three procedures, frozen sections are recommended, as they can undergo routine histopathology, immunohistochemistry, and molecular analysis. [20]

5.2. Cytology

Cytological evaluation reveals the phenotypes of infiltrating cells in the vitreous. The vitreous specimen is centrifuged and cells are smeared onto glass slides, and then immersed in 95% ethanol for Papanicolaou (Pap) staining or left to dry for Giemsa staining. [20]

The reported sensitivity of cytology in the detection of intraocular malignancy ranges from 31% to 66.7%. This relatively low yield may be due to the presence of immune cells, necrotic cells, fibrin, and debris in the specimen, which may confound the examination. [31] Other reasons include small sample volumes with a low number of malignant cells, inadequate preparation of the sample, and previous administration of corticosteroids. [20]

Cytologic evaluation may also be used to distinguish between a malignant process and an inflammatory disease. An example of an inflammatory etiology that may be diagnosed with the aid of cytology is sarcoidosis. Kinoshita et al. demonstrated multinucleated giant cells in the vitreous in 85.7% of cases and lymphocytes and epithelioid cells in all cases of intraocular sarcoidosis. [32]

An advanced technique for cytology is the use of cell blocks. They are superior to cell smears since cells are accumulated by centrifugation and stored as paraffin blocks. The large number of cells in a compacted area of one section on a slide glass as opposed to sparse cells on a smear leads to a more accurate diagnosis. Paraffin sections also have the advantage of being used for immunocytochemical diagnosis and clonal analysis, such as amplification by PCR of the immunoglobulin heavy chain gene. [33]

5.3. Microbiological analysis

Microbiological cultures are considered the "gold standard" for diagnosis of infectious uveitis. There are different types of media for isolation of the causative agent, including blood agar (for gram-positive or fastidious gram-negative bacteria [34]), MacConkey agar (for most gram-negative rods [34]), and Brucella agar for bacterial infections; Sabouraud dextrose agar for pathogenic fungi and yeast; and shell vial culture for viral infections. Along with the culture, the sample is sent for Gram staining and antibiotic sensitivity tests. [20]

Some fastidious organisms, such as *Proprionibacterium acnes* and fungi require holding the culture for at least 1 month to avoid missing their diagnosis. [21]

The sensitivity of culture after diagnostic vitrectomy for diagnosis of chronic infectious uveitis has been reported between 16.7% and 96%. [21] In cases of acute endophthalmitis, the sensitivity of microbiological cultures and stains was shown to be 40-70%. [35] Higher yields are reported with vitreous rather than aqueous samples. [36] Processing both diluted and undiluted vitreous samples increases the sensitivity of vitreous cultures to 57.4%. [37]

The yield of positive cultures from vitreous samples is usually low in cases of fungal endophthalmitis. In a retrospective study by Tanaka et al., positive cultures were only found in 38% of vitreous specimens in patients with endogenous fungal endophthalmitis. [38]

While the utility of Gram stains is limited in comparison with culture (data from the Endophthalmitis Vitrectomy Study showed a yield of 66% for culture and 41% for Gram stain for patients undergoing vitrectomy [35]), they are useful for rapid initial diagnosis of intraocular infection and can help the clinician choose the appropriate antibiotic for the organism prior to culture results.

5.4. Molecular analysis

Molecular analysis of a vitreous specimen is used for two main indications: 1) to diagnose PIOL 2) to detect the DNA of microorganisms in cases of infectious uveitis.

The techniques currently in use for molecular analysis include PCR, an in vitro technique used to amplify small quantities of nucleic acid into analytic amounts [39] and microdissection, which allows the selection and molecular analysis of malignant or atypical lymphoid cells from vitreous samples with a small amount of preserved cells. [31]

In cases of infectious uveitis, several PCR techniques may be used. Over the years new modifications to the basic method, such as real-time PCR and multiplex PCR have been developed. Real-time PCR allows for the characterization of an active infection versus low-grade pathogenicity by quantifying the number of pathogen genomes in a sample. Multiplex PCR allows for the amplification and detection of a number of different sequences at the same time (such as two infectious agents from a single sample). [40]

The addition of PCR to microbiological analysis has been shown to increase the diagnostic sensitivity from 48% to more than 80%. [41] Prior short-term use of intravitreal antibiotics does not affect its ability to amplify DNA. In one series of patients with postoperative endophthalmits treated with intravitreal antibiotics, PCR of vitreal specimens identified the causative organism in 10 of 16 patients (62%) versus only 3 (18%) with culture only. [42]

As the causative organism is not always known or suspected, a PCR technique that targets a specific microorganism is not always feasible. In such cases eubacterial PCR may be used. It targets the 16S ribosomal DNA (rRNA) common to all bacteria, thereby identifying a wider range of pathogens. [42-44] A similar approach detects the fungal genome in ocular fluids using probes that target the 18S rRNA present in the *Candida* and *Aspergillus* species, and probes that target the 28S rRNA also found in other species, including *Cryptococcus, Trichophyton, Mucor, Penicillium,* and *Pichia.* [45]

For PIOL diagnosis, PCR is used to detect monoclonality within the variable region of the third complementary determining region (CDR3) in the immunoglobulin heavy chain gene of malignant B cells. Single-band detection of immunoglobulin heavy chain rearrangement can be useful in PIOL. [20] In a study by Baehring et al., PCR was 64% sensitive for PIOL and identified immunoglobulin heavy chain gene rearrangements in four samples that were classified as negative for lymphoma based on cytopathology and flow cytometry. Cytology had 24% sensitivity and flow cytometry had a sensitivity of 36%. [46] In addition, PCR may be used to detect bcl-2 gene translocations in PIOL that were shown to occur in younger patients, suggesting a more aggressive treatment approach. [47]

5.5. Flow cytometry

Flow cytometry is a diagnostic technique that allows for simultaneous analysis of several different cell surface markers. It involves centrifuging diluted vitreous and re-suspension in cell culture medium. The cells are then counted and stained with antibodies to detect cellular surface markers that identify leukocytes. [20]

It has been shown to be useful in the diagnosis of PIOL. [16] It relies on the fact that most PIOLs are composed of monoclonal populations of B-lymphocytes that stain positively for B cell markers (CD19, CD20, CD22) and have restricted expression of κ or λ chains [48]

Davis et al [49] correlated different flow cytometric markers with lymphoma, infection, and idiopathic uveitis. They found that the most sensitive marker for lymphoma was a κ:λ ratio ≥3 or ≤0.6, while CD22 and CD20 were specific but not sensitive for lymphoma. For infection they found that the CD8, CD14, and CD11c markers that indicate monocytes and cytotoxic CD8$^+$ T lymphocytes were specific, but not sensitive. A CD4:CD8 ratio of ≥4 was highly sensitive and specific for inflammatory uveitis.

5.6. Cytokine measurement

B-cell malignancies can secrete high levels of interleukin-10 (IL-10), an immunosuppressive cytokine. Inflammatory conditions are associated with high levels of interleukin-6 (IL-6), a proinflammatory cytokine. [50, 51] IL-10 in PIOL tends to be high, with IL-10:IL-6 ratios greater than 1.0 being suggestive of the disease. This ratio may serve as a useful adjunctive test in the diagnosis of suspected PIOL, while also showing whether there is a significant response to treatment. [31]

Cassoux et al [52] found that mean IL-10 values were 2205.5 pg/mL in the vitreous and 543.4 pg/mL in the aqueous humor in patients with PIOL, while in uveitis patients mean values were 26.6 pg/mL in the vitreous and 21.9 pg/mL in the aqueous. This difference was highly significant.

Since the measurement of cytokine levels is fairly easy, measurement of IL-10 and IL-6 levels is recommended for patients with suspected PIOL. [20]

5.7. Antibody measurement

This indirect method of diagnosing infection is often negative early in the course of the disease as well as in immunocompromised patients. [31] Intraocular-specific antibody secretion has been shown to confirm the etiology in 23-32% of cases. [53, 54]

A helpful concept in antibody measurement is the Goldmann-Witmer coefficient (GWC). It can be calculated to compare intraocular antibody production with serum antibody levels. A ratio of greater than 1.0 is abnormal and ratios of 2-3 are considered significant. [55] Its accuracy has been shown in the case of toxoplasmosis. [56] Errera et al have shown that GWC testing had better sensitivity than PCR in ocular toxoplasmosis, especially when the test was carried out in younger patients with quiet eyes, with smaller sized chorioretinal lesions. In contrast, they have shown that this test was not helpful in viral retinitis in comparison to PCR, as the sensitivity and positive predictive value (PPV) were lower for GWC. [57]

6. Selected examples

6.1. Infectious etiologies

6.1.1. Bacterial and fungal endophthalmitis

In cases of suspected bacterial or fungal endophthalmitis, Gram stain and culture (aerobic, anerobic, and fungal) of the vitreous sample are performed in order to identify the causative organisms and their susceptibilities.

As mentioned above, PCR analysis of aqueous and vitreous fluid have also been applied in case series of patients with acute and delayed postoperative endophthalmitis, sometimes with better detection of the causative agent than cultures.

6.1.2. Mycobacterium tuberculosis

Diagnosis of ocular tuberculosis (TB) is possible with the use of various tests for the detection of systemic TB, including chest radiography, Purified Protein Derivative (PPD) tuberculin skin test, Interferon Gamma Release assays (IGRA), and analyses of extraocular sites. [58, 59] Intraocular fluid analysis may help.

Traditional fluid analysis with Ziehl-Neelsen staining and culture on Lowenstein-Jensen medium is not ideal, as the former has low yields and the latter takes up to 6-8 weeks, limiting its clinical utility. [58, 59] The yield of PCR analysis of aqueous and vitreous fluid has been shown to range from 37.7% to 72% in a series of Indian patients. [60-62] It was shown that 77-80% of PCR-positive patients in these series were PPD positive, and 90-100% of PCR-positive patients who were treated with antitubercular treatment had resolution of inflammation. Similar rates were shown by a Mexican group, [63] where PCR testing in 22 patients with a known diagnosis of TB uveitis showed a yield of 77.2%. All patients improved with antitubercular treatment.

6.1.3. Toxoplasma gondii

While diagnosis of ocular toxoplasmosis is typically made by a characteristic clinical presentation and supported by positive serology, there are cases that pose a diagnostic dilemma in which an invasive ocular diagnostic procedure may be needed. For example, in immunocompromised and elderly patients the disease may mimic viral necrotizing retinitis. [64, 65]

Culture of *T. gondii* from the vitreous may be lengthy and ranges from 2 to 23 days for positive cultures. [66] The rapid detection of toxoplasmosis DNA using PCR techniques on aqueous fluid has a yield of 13% to 55% according to literature, with positive results occurring more often with larger chorioretinal lesions, immunosuppressed patients, and active anterior segment inflammation. [21] Antibody levels in the aqueous may supplement PCR results by calculating the GWC, as described above. In one series, calculation of the aqueous GWC for toxoplasmosis antibody at the onset of clinical manifestation had a yield of 57%, rising to 70% after 3 weeks. [67]

The utility of GWC is decreased in immunocompromised patients. In one series of 34 immunocompetent patients with negative PCR tests for toxoplasmosis, 25 had a positive GWC, whereas none of the immunocompromised patients exhibited a positive test. [56] In a similar fashion, another series showed 93% positivity with use of this test in immunocompetent patients, in comparison with a yield of only 57% in immunocompromised patients. [68]

While these results deal with aqueous analysis, less data appears in the literature regarding diagnostic vitrectomy for this purpose. Available data shows a trend towards improved yields for PCR from vitreous specimens. [21]

6.1.4. Viral retinitis

The diagnosis of infectious viral retinitis caused by herpes simplex virus (HSV), cytomegalovirus (CMV), or varicella zoster virus (VZV) is not always straightforward. As with the other infectious entities just mentioned, growth on culture may take a long time. PCR analysis of aqueous and vitreous fluid plays an important role thanks to its high sensitivity, low false-positive rates, and the rapidity of the assay. [69, 70]

The sensitivities of PCR for VZV, HSV, and CMV were reported to exceed 90%, with specificities in excess of 95%. [39] Knox et al. performed PCR on specimens from 38 eyes of 37 patients with an inflammation of unknown etiology suggestive of an infectious posterior segment disease. In 24 of these cases CMV, HSV, or VZV were detected. [71] Sugita et al. collected 68 aqueous humor samples and 43 vitreous fluid samples from 100 patients with uveitis. The samples were assayed for human herpes viruses using multiplex PCR and real-time PCR. Out of 16 patients with ARN, either HSV1, HSV2, or VZV genomes were detected. In another 10 patients with anterior uveitis with iris atrophy, the VZV genome was detected. Epstein-Barr virus was detected in 17% of samples, and (CMV) was detected in three patients with anterior uveitis of immunocompetent patients and in one immunocompromised CMV retinitis patient. [72]

As was shown above for toxoplasmosis, calculation of the GWC may also be of use for HSV, VZV, and CMV, although variable results have been reported in the literature. In one series of immunocompromised patients with posterior uveitis and panuveitis, analysis of an aqueous sample demonstrated a detection rate of 94% for PCR aimed for the detection of CMV and VZV versus only 18% with GWC. [73] Another series demonstrated an identification of 92% of HSV-associated and 87.5% of VZV-associated infectious uveitis using GWC, in comparison with 54% of HSV and 75% VZV cases that were identified using PCR. [74]

6.2. Non-infectious inflammatory conditions

6.2.1. Sarcoidosis

The frequency of sarcoidosis involving the posterior segment varies in different series. One group reported that as many as 89% of patients with ocular sarcoidosis demonstrated posterior segment involvement, with vitritis as the most common manifestation, present in 69% of these patients. [75] As the manifestations of sarcoidosis are varied, a diagnosis of this inflammatory entity is not always straightforward, and may require an invasive procedure such as diagnostic pars plana vitrectomy.

An increased CD4+ helper T-cell type 1 lymphocyte subset in bronchoalveolar lavage (BAL) fluid and a high CD4/CD8 ratio are helpful for the diagnosis of sarcoidosis. [76] Kojima et al. demonstrated that this ratio may also be applied for vitreous specimens, when a CD4/CD8 ratio of vitreous-infiltrating lymphocytes greater than 3.5 provided a diagnosis of ocular sarcoidosis with a sensitivity of 100% and a specificity of 96.3% (in comparison with a sensitivity of 53% and specificity of 94% in analysis of BAL fluid). [77]

6.3. Neoplastic processes

6.3.1. Primary intraocular lymphoma

PIOL is considered one of the masquerade syndromes, or diseases that mimic inflammatory conditions in presentation, leading to a diagnostic dilemma. [78] When the diagnosis of a neoplastic process such as PIOL is suspected, reaching a diagnosis is of utmost importance in terms of prognosis and the choice of treatment.

A definitive tissue diagnosis is required to make the diagnosis of PIOL. If lymphoma is identified from a lumbar puncture, an invasive diagnostic ocular procedure may not be required. If, on the other hand, lumbar puncture results are inconclusive and neuroimaging is not consistent with CNS lymphoma in a patient with a high index of suspicion for PIOL, invasive diagnostic procedures are appropriate. [3]

Histologic identification of malignant lymphoid cells is the gold standard for diagnosing PIOL. [3] As stated above, it is pertinent to communicate with the pathologist before the procedure, as any delay in delivery of the sample may result in death of acquired cells.

The characteristic features of PIOL using microscopic analyses include large atypical lymphoid cells with scarce cytoplasm, prominent nucleoli, frequently large segmented nuclei, and a high nuclear to cytoplasm ratio. [3] Cytology has a sensitivity ranging from 31% to 66.7% for detecting intraocular malignancy, and one report showed a sensitivity of 83.3% for detecting PIOL. [31, 49] In addition to cytology, immunohistochemistry, cytokine analysis, flow cytometry, and gene rearrangements by PCR are also performed on the specimens. [3]

6.3.2. Tumor metastasis

Tumor metastasis is the most common cause of intraocular malignancy in adults. [78] While their typical appearance and preexisting history of cancer typically lead to diagnosis, uveal metastases masquerading as intraocular inflammation have been reported. [21]

A few cases were reported on the use of aqueous sampling for cytology which led to the diagnosis of metastases masquerading as anterior uveitis. [79-84] Of patients undergoing diagnostic vitrectomy for uveitis of unknown cause, detection of metastasis from cytology results was rare in the literature, [11, 85, 86] with only one case reported in each of these series. In case reports of patients with the rare occurrence of tumors metastatic to the retina and vitreous, these conditions present as intermediate uveitis, vitreous hemorrhage, or retinal vasculitis with vitreous cytology and retinal biopsy assisting in diagnosis if no primary malignancy is identified. [21]

In a series of 159 cases by Shields et al, [87] transocular fine needle aspiration (FNA) biopsy led to an adequate sample collection in 88% of cases, with a sensitivity rate of 100% and specificity rate of 98%, leading to diagnosis of intraocular malignancies such as uveal melanoma, uveal metastasis, retinoblastoma, lymphoma, and leukemia. In another series of 39 patients with uveal metastasis undergoing ocular biopsy of the tumor, 25 G vitrectomy had a yield of 100% for cytologic diagnosis. It indicated the site of origin in 24 out of 27 patients without a known primary tumor. [88]

7. Summary

Diagnostic procedures in ophthalmology have gone a long way from the early days of pars plana vitrectomy, when instrumentation and diagnostic methods were limited and the amount of entities that could be diagnosed by invasive methods was restricted.

As this chapter has shown, the approach to a patient with a cryptic diagnosis, a rapidly deteriorating disease, or treatment failure has changed in the last decades and ophthalmologists now have in their arsenal a battery of tools to help in the diagnosis of cases that were once considered unsolvable or untreatable.

Author details

Roy Schwartz and Zohar Habot-Wilner*

*Address all correspondence to: zoharhw@tlvmc.gov.il

Ophthalmology division, Tel-Aviv Medical Center, the Sackler Faculty of Medicine, Tel Aviv University, Israel

References

[1] Michels RG, Machemer R, Mueller-Jensen K (1974) Vitreous surgery: history and current concepts. Ophthal Surg 5:13-59.

[2] Engel HM, Green WR, Michels RG, et al. (1981) Diagnostic vitrectomy. Retina 1:121-49.

[3] Hwang CS, Yeh S, Bergstrom CS (2014) Diagnostic vitrectomy for primary intraocular lymphoma: when, why, how? Int Ophthalmol Clin 54:155-71. doi: 10.1097/IIO. 0000000000000022

[4] Durand M (1997) Microbiologic factors and visual outcome in the Endophthalmitis Vitrectomy Study. Am J Ophthalmol 124:127-130.

[5] Kanoff J, Sobrin L (2011) New diagnosis and treatment paradigms in acute retinal necrosis. Int Ophthalmol Clin 51:25-31. doi: 10.1097/IIO.0b013e31822d6864

[6] Nussenblatt RB, Whitcup SW (2010) Uveitis: fundamentals and clinical practice, 4th ed. St. Louis: Mosby Elsevier.

[7] Trivedi D, Denniston AK, Murray PI (2011) Safety profile of anterior chamber paracentesis performed at the slit lamp. Clin Exp Ophthalmol 39:725-728. doi: 10.1111/j. 1442-9071.2011.02565.x

[8] Augsburger JJ (1990) Invasive diagnostic techniques for uveitis and simulating conditions. Trans Pa Acad Ophthalmol Otolaryngol 42:964-971.

[9] Lobo A, Lightman S (2003) Vitreous aspiration needle tap in the diagnosis of intraocular inflammation. Ophthalmology 110:595-599. doi: 10.1016/S0161-6420(02)01895-X

[10] Forster RK, Abbott RL, Gelender H (1980) Management of infectious endophthalmitis. Ophthalmology 87:313-319.

[11] Verbraeken H (1996) Diagnostic vitrectomy and chronic uveitis. Graefes Arch Clin Exp Ophthalmol 234 Suppl:S2-S7. doi: 10.1007/BF02343040

[12] Bovey EH, Herbort CP (2000) Vitrectomy in the management of uveitis. Ocul Immunol Inflamm 8:285-291.

[13] Carroll DM, Franklin RM (1981) Vitreous biopsy in uveitis of unknown cause. Retina 1:245-251. doi: 10.1097/00006982-198101030-00022

[14] Akpek EK, Ahmed I, Hochberg FH, et al. (1999) Intraocular-central nervous system lymphoma: clinical features, diagnosis, and outcomes. Ophthalmology 106:1805-1810. doi: 10.1016/S0161-6420(99)90341-X

[15] Mruthyunjaya P, Jumper JM, McCallum R, et al. (2002) Diagnostic yield of vitrectomy in eyes with suspected posterior segment infection or malignancy. Ophthalmology 109:1123-1129. doi: 10.1016/S0161-6420(02)01033-3

[16] Zaldivar RA, Martin DF, Holden JT, Grossniklaus HE (2004) Primary intraocular lymphoma: clinical, cytologic, and flow cytometric analysis. Ophthalmology 111:1762-1767. doi: 10.1016/j.ophtha.2004.03.021

[17] De Groot-Mijnes JDF, Rothova A (2006) Diagnostic testing of vitrectomy specimens. Am J Ophthalmol 141:982. doi: 10.1016/j.ajo.2006.01.028

[18] Margolis R, Brasil OFM, Lowder CY, et al. (2007) Vitrectomy for the diagnosis and management of uveitis of unknown cause. Ophthalmology 114:1893-1897. doi: 10.1016/j.ophtha.2007.01.038

[19] Oahalou A, Schellekens PAWJF, de Groot-Mijnes JD, Rothova A (2014) Diagnostic pars plana vitrectomy and aqueous analyses in patients with uveitis of unknown cause. Retina 34:108-114. doi: 10.1097/IAE.0b013e31828e6985

[20] Ryan SJ, Schachat AP, Wilkinson CP, Hinton DR, Sadda S, Wiedemann P (Eds.) (2006) Retina, 5th edition, Elsevier.

[21] Jeroudi A, Yeh S (2014) Diagnostic vitrectomy for infectious uveitis. Int Ophthalmol Clin 54:173-197. doi: 10.1097/IIO.0000000000000017

[22] Feng H, Adelman RA (2014) Cataract formation following vitreoretinal procedures. Clin Ophthalmol 8:1957-1965. doi: 10.2147/OPTH.S68661

[23] Thompson JT (2004) The role of patient age and intraocular gas use in cataract progression after vitrectomy for macular holes and epiretinal membranes. Am J Ophthalmol 137:250-257. doi: 10.1016/j.ajo.2003.09.020

[24] Vela JI, Rosello N, Diaz-Cascajosa J, et al. (2010) Combined retinal detachment and candida chorioretinitis. Case Reports 2010:bcr0120102648-bcr0120102648. doi: 10.1136/bcr.01.2010.2648

[25] Jalil A, Ho WO, Charles S, et al. (2013) Iatrogenic retinal breaks in 20-G versus 23-G pars plana vitrectomy. Graefe's Arch Clin Exp Ophthalmol 251:1463-1467. doi: 10.1007/s00417-013-2299-2

[26] Lau CH, Missotten T, Salzmann J, Lightman SL (2007) Acute retinal necrosis. Features, management, and outcomes. Ophthalmology. doi: 10.1016/j.ophtha.2006.08.037

[27] Chang S (2006) LXII Edward Jackson lecture: open angle glaucoma after vitrectomy. Am J Ophthalmol. doi: 10.1016/j.ajo.2006.02.014

[28] Retina and Vitreous, section 12. Basic and Clinical Science Course (BCSC). American Academy of Ophthalmology 2012-2013.

[29] Bechrakis NE, Foerster MH, Bornfeld N (2002) Biopsy in indeterminate intraocular tumors. Ophthalmology 109:235-242. doi: 10.1016/S0161-6420(01)00931-9

[30] Johnston RL, Tufail A, Lightman S, et al. (2004) Retinal and choroidal biopsies are helpful in unclear uveitis of suspected infectious or malignant origin. Ophthalmology 111:522-528. doi: 10.1016/j.ophtha.2002.10.002

[31] Margolis R (2008) Diagnostic vitrectomy for the diagnosis and management of posterior uveitis of unknown etiology. Curr Opin Ophthalmol 19:218-224. doi: 10.1097/ICU.0b013e3282fc261d

[32] Kinoshita Y, Takasu K, Adachi Y, et al. (2012) Diagnostic utility of vitreous humor fluid cytology for intraocular sarcoidosis: a clinicopathologic study of 7 cases. Diagn Cytopathol 40:210-213. doi: 10.1002/dc.21540

[33] Matsuo T, Ichimura K (2012) Immunocytochemical diagnosis as inflammation by vitrectomy cell blocks in patients with vitreous opacity. Ophthalmology 119:827-837. doi: 10.1016/j.ophtha.2011.10.020

[34] Harvey RA, Champe PC, Fisher BD (2007) Lippincott's illustrated reviews: microbiology, 2nd edition (Lippincott's Illustrated Reviews Series). Lippincott Williams & Wilkins.

[35] Han DP, Wisniewski SR, Kelsey SF, et al. (1999) Microbiologic yields and complication rates of vitreous needle aspiration versus mechanized vitreous biopsy in the Endophthalmitis Vitrectomy Study. Retina 19:98-102.

[36] Okhravi N, Adamson P, Carroll N, et al. (2000) PCR-based evidence of bacterial involvement in eyes with suspected intraocular infection. Investig Ophthalmol Vis Sci 41:3474-3479.

[37] Donahue SP, Kowalski RP, Jewart BH, Friberg TR (1993) Vitreous cultures in suspected endophthalmitis. Biopsy or vitrectomy? Ophthalmology 100:452-455.

[38] Tanaka M, Kobayashi Y, Takebayashi H, et al. (2001) Analysis of predisposing clinical and laboratory findings for the development of endogenous fungal endophthalmitis. A retrospective 12-year study of 79 eyes of 46 patients. Retina 21:203-209. doi: 10.1097/00006982-200106000-00001

[39] Van Gelder RN (2003) Cme review: polymerase chain reaction diagnostics for posterior segment disease. Retina 23:445-452. doi: 10.1097/00006982-200308000-00001

[40] Yeung SN, Butler A, Mackenzie PJ (2009) Applications of the polymerase chain reaction in clinical ophthalmology. Can J Ophthalmol 44:23-30. doi: 10.3129/I08-161

[41] Garweg JG, Wanner D, Sarra GM, et al. (2006) The diagnostic yield of vitrectomy specimen analysis in chronic idiopathic endogenous uveitis. Eur J Ophthalmol 16:588-594.

[42] Chiquet C, Lina G, Benito Y, et al. (2007) Polymerase chain reaction identification in aqueous humor of patients with postoperative endophthalmitis. J Cataract Refract Surg 33:635-641. doi: 10.1016/j.jcrs.2006.12.017

[43] Chiquet C, Cornut PL, Benito Y, et al. (2008) Eubacterial PCR for bacterial detection and identification in 100 acute postcataract surgery endophthalmitis. Investig Ophthalmol Vis Sci 49:1971-1978. doi: 10.1167/iovs.07-1377

[44] Chiquet C, Maurin M, Thuret G, et al. (2009) Analysis of Diluted Vitreous Samples from Vitrectomy Is Useful in Eyes with Severe Acute Postoperative Endophthalmitis. Ophthalmology. doi: 10.1016/j.ophtha.2009.06.007

[45] Ogawa M, Sugita S, Watanabe K, et al. (2012) Novel diagnosis of fungal endophthalmitis by broad-range real-time PCR detection of fungal 28S ribosomal DNA. Graefe's Arch Clin Exp Ophthalmol 250:1877-1883. doi: 10.1007/s00417-012-2015-7

[46] Baehring JM, Androudi S, Longtine JJ, et al. (2005) Analysis of clonal immunoglobulin heavy chain rearrangements in ocular lymphoma. Cancer 104:591-597. doi: 10.1002/cncr.21191

[47] Wallace DJ, Shen D, Reed GF, et al. (2006) Detection of the bcl-2 t(14;18) translocation and proto-oncogene expression in primary intraocular lymphoma. Investig Ophthalmol Vis Sci 47:2750-2756. doi: 10.1167/iovs.05-1312

[48] Chan CC, Wallace DJ (2004) Intraocular lymphoma: update on diagnosis and management. Cancer Control 11:285-295.

[49] Davis JL, Miller DM, Ruiz P (2005) Diagnostic testing of vitrectomy specimens. Am J Ophthalmol 140:822-829. doi: 10.1016/j.ajo.2005.05.032

[50] Wolf LA, Reed GF, Buggage RR, et al. (2003) Vitreous cytokine levels. Ophthalmology 110:1671-1672. doi: 10.1016/S0161-6420(03)00811-X

[51] Merle-Béral H, Davi F, Cassoux N, et al. (2004) Biological diagnosis of primary intraocular lymphoma. Br J Haematol 124:469-473.

[52] Cassoux N, Giron A, Bodaghi B, et al. (2007) IL-10 measurement in aqueous humor for screening patients with suspicion of primary intraocular lymphoma. Investig Ophthalmol Vis Sci 48:3253-3259. doi: 10.1167/iovs.06-0031

[53] De Groot-Mijnes JDF, De Visser L, Rothova A, et al. (2006) Rubella virus is associated with Fuchs heterochromic iridocyclitis. Am J Ophthalmol. doi: 10.1016/j.ajo.2005.07.078

[54] Rothova A, de Boer JH, Ten Dam-van Loon NH, et al. (2008) Usefulness of aqueous humor analysis for the diagnosis of posterior uveitis. Ophthalmology 115:306-311. doi: 10.1016/j.ophtha.2007.05.014

[55] Damato EM, Angi M, Romano MR, et al. (2012) Vitreous analysis in the management of uveitis. Mediators Inflamm. doi: 10.1155/2012/863418

[56] Fardeau C, Romand S, Rao NA, et al. (2002) Diagnosis of toxoplasmic retinochoroiditis with atypical clinical features. Am J Ophthalmol 134:196-203. doi: 10.1016/S0002-9394(02)01500-3

[57] Errera MH, Goldschmidt P, Batellier L, et al. (2011) Real-time polymerase chain reaction and intraocular antibody production for the diagnosis of viral versus toxoplasmic infectious posterior uveitis. Graefe's Arch Clin Exp Ophthalmol 249:1837-1846. doi: 10.1007/s00417-011-1724-7

[58] Gupta V, Gupta A, Rao NA (2007) Intraocular tuberculosis-an update. Surv Ophthalmol 52:561-587. doi: 10.1016/j.survophthal.2007.08.015

[59] Vasconcelos-Santos DV, Zierhut M, Rao NA (2009) Strengths and weaknesses of diagnostic tools for tuberculous uveitis diagnostic tools for tuberculous uveitis. Ocul Immunol Inflamm 17:351-355.

[60] Arora SK, Gupta V, Gupta A, et al. (1999) Diagnostic efficacy of polymerase chain reaction in granulomatous uveitis. Tuber Lung Dis 79:229-233. doi: 10.1054/tuld. 1999.0210

[61] Gupta V, Arora S, Gupta A, et al. (1998) Management of presumed intraocular tuberculosis: possible role of the polymerase chain reaction. Acta Ophthalmol Scand 76:679-682.

[62] Gupta A, Gupta V, Arora S, et al. (2001) PCR-positive tubercular retinal vasculitis: clinical characteristics and management. Retina 21:435-444. doi: 10.1097/00006982-200110000-00004

[63] Ortega-Larrocea G, Bobadilla-Del-Valle M, Ponce-De-León A, Sifuentes-Osornio J (2003) Nested polymerase chain reaction for Mycobacterium tuberculosis DNA detection in aqueous and vitreous of patients with uveitis. Arch Med Res 34:116-119. doi: 10.1016/S0188-4409(02)00467-8

[64] Johnson MW, Greven GM, Jaffe GJ, et al. (1997) Atypical, severe toxoplasmic retinochoroiditis in elderly patients. Ophthalmology 104:48-57.

[65] Moshfeghi DM, Dodds EM, Couto CA, et al. (2004) Diagnostic approaches to severe, atypical toxoplasmosis mimicking acute retinal necrosis. Ophthalmology 111:716-725. doi: 10.1016/j.ophtha.2003.07.004

[66] Miller D, Davis J, Rosa R, et al. (2000) Utility of tissue culture for detection of Toxoplasma gondii in vitreous humor of patients diagnosed with toxoplasmic retinochoroiditis. J Clin Microbiol 38:3840-3842.

[67] Garweg JG, Jacquier P, Boehnke M (2000) Early aqueous humor analysis in patients with human ocular toxoplasmosis. J Clin Microbiol 38:996-1001.

[68] Rothova A, de Boer JH, ten Dam-van Loon NH, et al. (2008) Usefulness of aqueous humor analysis for the diagnosis of posterior uveitis. Ophthalmology 115:306-311. doi: 10.1016/j.ophtha.2007.05.014

[69]   Fox GM, Crouse CA, Chuang EL, et al. (1991) Detection of herpesvirus DNA in vitreous and aqueous specimens by the polymerase chain reaction. Arch Ophthalmol 109:266-271. doi: 10.1001/archopht.1991.01080020112054

[70]   Pendergast SD, Werner J, Drevon A, Wiedbrauk DL (2000) Absence of herpesvirus DNA by polymerase chain reaction in ocular fluids obtained from immunocompetent patients. Retina 20:389-393. doi: 10.1097/00006982-200007000-00012

[71]   Knox CM, Chandler D, Short GA, Margolis TP (1998) Polymerase chain reaction-based assays of vitreous samples for the diagnosis of viral retinitis: use in diagnostic dilemmas. Ophthalmology 105:37-45. doi: 10.1016/S0161-6420(98)71127-2

[72]   Sugita S, Shimizu N, Watanabe K, et al. (2008) Use of multiplex PCR and real-time PCR to detect human herpes virus genome in ocular fluids of patients with uveitis. Br J Ophthalmol 92:928-932. doi: 10.1136/bjo.2007.133967

[73]   Westeneng AC, Rothova A, de Boer JH, de Groot-Mijnes JDF (2007) Infectious uveitis in immunocompromised patients and the diagnostic value of polymerase chain reaction and Goldmann-Witmer coefficient in aqueous analysis. Am J Ophthalmol 144:781-785. doi: 10.1016/j.ajo.2007.06.034

[74]   De Groot-Mijnes JDF, Rothova A, Van Loon AM, et al. (2006) Polymerase chain reaction and goldmann-witmer coefficient analysis are complimentary for the diagnosis of infectious uveitis. Am J Ophthalmol 141:313-318. doi: 10.1016/j.ajo.2005.09.017

[75]   Khalatbari D, Stinnett S, McCallum RM, Jaffe GJ (2004) Demographic-related variations in posterior segment ocular sarcoidosis. Ophthalmology 111:357-362. doi: 10.1016/S0161-6420(03)00793-0

[76]   (1999) Statement on sarcoidosis. Joint Statement of the American Thoracic Society (ATS), the European Respiratory Society (ERS) and the World Association of Sarcoidosis and Other Granulomatous Disorders (WASOG) adopted by the ATS Board of Directors and by the ER. Am J Respir Crit Care Med 160:736-755. doi: 10.1164/ajrccm.160.2.ats4-99

[77]   Kojima K, Maruyama K, Inaba T, et al. (2012) The CD4/CD8 ratio in vitreous fluid is of high diagnostic value in sarcoidosis. Ophthalmology 119:2386-2392. doi: 10.1016/j.ophtha.2012.05.033

[78]   Read RW, Zamir E, Rao NA (2002) Neoplastic masquerade syndromes. Surv Ophthalmol 47:81-124. doi: 10.1016/S0039-6257(01)00305-8

[79]   Talegaonkar SK (1969) Anterior uveal tract metastasis as the presenting feature of bronchial carcinoma. Br J Ophthalmol 53:123-126.

[80]   Morgan WE, Malmgren RA, Albert DM (1970) Metastatic carcinoma of the ciliary body simulating uveitis. Diagnosis by cytologic examination of aqueous humor. Arch Ophthalmol 83:54-58.

[81] Denslow GT, Kielar RA (1978) Metastatic adenocarcinoma to the anterior uvea and increased carcinoembryonic antigen levels. Am J Ophthalmol 85:363-367.

[82] Scholz R, Green WR, Baranano EC, et al. (1983) Metastatic carcinoma to the iris. Diagnosis by aqueous paracentesis and response to irradiation and chemotherapy. Ophthalmology 90:1524-1527.

[83] Takahashi T, Oda Y, Chiba T, et al. (1984) Metastatic carcinoma of the iris and ciliary body simulating iridocyclitis. Ophthalmologica 188:266-272. doi: 10.1159/000309373

[84] Woog JJ, Chess J, Albert DM, et al. (1984) Metastatic carcinoma of the iris simulating iridocyclitis. Br J Ophthalmol 68:167-173. doi: 10.1136/bjo.68.3.167

[85] Priem H, Verbraeken H, de Laey JJ (1993) Diagnostic problems in chronic vitreous inflammation. Graefes Arch Clin Exp Ophthalmol 231:453-456. doi: 10.1007/BF02044231

[86] Palexas GN, Green WR, Goldberg MF, Ding Y (1995) Diagnostic pars plana vitrectomy report of a 21-year retrospective study. Trans Am Ophthalmol Soc 93:281-308; discussion 308-314.

[87] Shields JA, Shields CL, Ehya H, et al. (1993) Fine-needle aspiration biopsy of suspected intraocular tumors. The 1992 Urwick Lecture. Ophthalmology 100:1677-1684. doi: 10.1097/00004397-199303330-00012

[88] Konstantinidis L, Rospond-Kubiak I, Zeolite I, et al. (2014) Management of patients with uveal metastases at the Liverpool Ocular Oncology Centre. Br J Ophthalmol 98:92-98. doi: 10.1136/bjophthalmol-2013-303519

3

Surgical Management of Epiretinal Membrane

Miltiadis K. Tsilimbaris, Chrysanthi Tsika,
George Kontadakis and Athanassios Giarmoukakis

Abstract

Epiretinal membranes (ERMs) are contractile membranes that occur on the inner surface of the retina and can lead to significant visual impairment when located at the central retina. Recent advances in vitreoretinal surgery have greatly improved the safety and efficacy of microsurgical intervention at the retinal surface level. Today, vitrectomy and membrane peels are considered the treatment of choice for most patients with ERMs that create significant visual symptoms. Nevertheless, possible complications such as accelerated cataract formation, recurrence of ERM and retinal detachment may withhold the choice of surgical intervention. Additionally, in some cases, simple observation may be advised. In view of surgery, controversies regarding techniques such as those related to an internal limiting membrane peel and the use of dye still exist. In this chapter, we cover current surgical techniques for ERM removal, their expected results, possible complications, as well as a guide for possible case selection.

Keywords: Epiretinal membrane, surgical management, patient selection

1. Introduction

1.1. Classification

The disease entity of epiretinal membrane (ERM) proliferation was first described in 1865 by Iwanoff [1]. It is caused by the proliferation of avascular cellular sheets on the inner retinal surface and along the internal limiting membrane (ILM), which possesses contractile properties and as a result, leads to variable visual symptoms and visual impairments, primarily due to the mechanical distortion of the macular area. The condition's variable effect on vision is determined primarily by the severity of the retinal distortion and the location of the membrane.

ERMs can be classified according to their underlying aetiology into: a) primary or idiopathic ERMs (iERMs) [2], when no underlying causative factor or ocular pathology can be associated with the membrane formation; b) secondary ERMs, which are commonly found in association with retinal breaks and retinal detachment (RD), RD surgical repair, laser photocoagulation, retinal cryopexy, proliferative vitreoretinopathy (PVR), retinal vascular diseases, intraocular inflammation and ocular trauma [3-7]. Additionally, international literature describes rare cases of secondary ERM formation associated with type-2 neurofibromatosis [8]. In addition to the etiological classification, Gass proposed a clinical classification of ERMs based on biomicroscopical findings [9], according to which ERMs can be differentiated into three grades:

a.   Grade 0 membranes or cellophane maculopathy. Translucent membranes not associated with retinal or visual distortion.

b.   Grade 1 membranes or crinkled cellophane maculopathy. Membranes causing an irregular wrinkling of the inner retinal surface due to the contraction of the overlying membrane. Increased vascular tortuosity and perimacular vessels being pulled toward the fovea are common findings.

c.   Grade 2 membranes or macular puckers. Opaque and thick membranes that cause profound retinal distortion and tractional phenomena. Cystic macular oedema, intraretinal haemorrhages, exudates, foveal ectopia and shallow localized retinal detachment can be accompanying findings in biomicroscopy.

2. Epidemiology and pathophysiology

Idiopathic membranes and membranes associated with RD or retinal tears, as well as their management, are the most prevalent clinical phenotypes of ERM proliferation [10]. The prevalence of iERM in the general population is estimated to be approximately 6 to 7% [11], with the disease's prevalence increasing significantly with age. Specifically, according to epidemiologic studies, the prevalence of ERM formation is increasing from 2% under the age of 60 years to 12 to 20% beyond the age of 70 [2, 10], while it is bilateral in 10 to 30% of cases [11-12]. Nevertheless, lower prevalence rates have been recorded in Chinese populations [13]. Moreover, histopathological findings suggest the presence of iERMs in 1.7 to 3.5% of autopsied eyes [12-14]. Regarding secondary ERMs, the disease incidence is 4 to 8% following surgical management of rhegmatogenous RD [15-16] and 1 to 2% following precautionary treatment of peripheral retinal breaks [17].

The proposed theories regarding the underlying pathophysiology of ERM formation have been controversial; furthermore, the exact origin and type of cells that make up different types of ERMs remains an area of debate [14, 18]. Nevertheless, the general consensus is that the primary cell component in iERMs is of glial origin, more recently called laminocytes, while secondary ERMs predominantly consist of different cell types that do not originate in the neuroretina, such as retinal pigment epithelial (RPE) cells, macrophages, myofibroblasts and fibrocytes, depending on the causative ocular pathology [19-20]. Posterior vitreous detachment (PVD), complete as well as partial, seems to play an important role in ERM pathogenesis. Specifically, it is well documented that PVD is present in up to 90% of eyes with iERMs and in fact, in all eyes with ERM formation associated with RD or retinal breaks [21]. It is therefore believed that glial cells from the neuroretina migrate through breaks in the ILM occurring during the PVD process and start to proliferate on the inner retinal surface, resulting in the formation of iERMs [18]. According to another theory, residual vitreous on the retinal surface following PVD may be related to the development of iERMs [22]. Nevertheless, iERM formation is also known to take place in eyes without PVD. In these cases, different theories have been proposed, including the migration of cells of glial origin through pre-existing ILM breaks or due to ILM thinning [23]; additionally, the vitreous traction theory proposes that astrocytic gliosis, commonly triggered by ischaemia and vitreous traction, can also occur in cases with partial or anomalous PVD (vitreoschisis), or even in the absence of PVD due to the coexistence of vitreous-retina attachment (complete or partial) with simultaneous vitreous movement, which is facilitated by the natural liquefying process of the vitreous, ultimately generating active vitreous traction and therefore, astrocytic gliosis [24]. On the other hand, the formation of secondary ERMs that develop in association with retinal breaks, RD, cryopexy and laser photocoagulation, most likely represents a form of mild PVR caused by the release of RPE cells into the vitreous cavity and their subsequent proliferation on the retinal surface [25]. In their recent work, Snead and colleagues [26], using surgically peeled membrane specimens and normal cadaver globes, determined the principal cell populations that characterize different types of ERMs, thus allowing for a clinical classification of ERMs based on their histopathological characteristics, which reflect different aetiologies. Specifically, they concluded that idiopathic ERMs are characterized by laminocytes and ILM, while the presence of laminocytes both on the ILM surface and the posterior hyaloid membrane (PHM) in cases of PVD raised the hypothesis that separation can likely occur due to the cellular activity of pre-existing laminocytes at the vitreoretinal interface. In ERMs, secondary to RD, retinal tears, PVR, trauma or intraocular inflammation, RPE cells, macrophages, lymphocytes and collagen were the primary cell components indicating that these ERMs most likely represent a tissue repair reaction. Furthermore, ERMs, secondary to PDR and vasoproliferative tumours, consisted mainly of capillaries and acellular stromal tissue, and were therefore characterized as neovascular ERMs, with hypoxia likely being the main stimulus for their formation.

In addition, recent studies implementing novel immunohistochemistry and proteomics techniques have attempted to elucidate the role of inflammatory cytokines and trophic factors in ERM development and proliferation. Basic fibroblast growth factor (bFGF) supports the survival and proliferation of glial cells and may play an important role in the ERM pathogenesis [27]. Harada et al. [28] encountered increased reactivity and expression of the bFGF in the majority of iERM and PDR-associated ERM cases studied. In accordance, similar results were reported by Chen et al. [29]. Other studies stressed the role of the nerve growth factor (NGF) and the transforming growth factors $\beta1$ and $\beta2$ (TGF$\beta1$ and TGF$\beta2$) in iERM formation and their subsequent contraction [30-31]. Authors suggested that these trophic factors possibly induce the differentiation of glial cells into myofibroblasts, granting ERMs their contractile properties [30-31]. Increased expression of the vascular endothelial growth factor (VEGF) has also been reported in iERMs, though its exact role in the disease pathogenesis still remains unknown [29, 32-33]. Furthermore, proteins such as apolipoprotein A-1, transthyretin, α-antitrypsin, serum albumin and interleukin-6 have also been proposed to participate in the pathogenesis of the disease [27, 34].

3. Natural course and associated symptoms

ERMs tend to remain stable or to present limited progression over time, with most patients experiencing mild or no symptoms following the initial diagnosis, indicating that membrane contraction possibly occurs at an early phase after its original formation and generally stabilizes thereafter. According to the findings of the population based "Blue Mountains Eye Study", epiretinal membrane progression was encountered in 28.6% of cases, stability was noticed in 38.8% of eyes, while 25.7% of cases regressed during a five-year follow-up period [35]. Accordingly, former studies have supported the non-progressive character of the disease [36-37], since only 10 to 25% of eyes seemed to show a significant decrease in visual acuity over time, with variable rates of progression [2, 9]. In fact, previous reports suggest that less than 5% of ERM cases present visual acuity of 20/200 or worse [38-39]. Moreover, rare cases of spontaneous ERM separation from the retina with associated visual improvement have also been documented [9, 40].

ERMs are symptomatic only if the macular or peri-macular area is involved. In its mildest forms, such as in cases of cellophane maculopathy, the disease is usually asymptomatic [38-39]. Symptomatic patients usually complain of decreased visual acuity (VA), metamorphopsia or vague visual disturbances. Other less common symptoms include micropsia and monocular diplopia [38-39]. In general terms, the extent of the visual effect of the disease is determined mainly by the degree of the induced retinal distortion, the position of the membrane in association to the macula, as well as its thickness and transparency. The decrease in VA can generally be attributed to the filtering effect of the ERM that prevents light from reaching the photoreceptors, the distortion of the retinal surface, as well as the macular oedema and the associated vitreoretinal traction due to incomplete PVD, if present. The distortion of the retinal surface due to ERM contraction, which in some cases can involve the entire retinal thickness, is the primary cause for metamorphopsia, which is usually the leading and most disturbing symptom of the disease.

4. Diagnosis

The diagnosis of the disease is primarily clinical, based on fundus biomicroscopy. In its mildest form, ERM is detected only as a mild glistening light reflex from the inner retina. Fundus examination or fundus photographs with a blue filter may facilitate visualization of very thin membranes [41]. In more advanced cases, wrinkling and/or striae of the retinal surface, as well as retinal vessel distortion may be noticed during examination. Usually, the membrane itself is invisible; nevertheless in advanced cases and particularly in cases of secondary membranes associated with retinal breaks and RD, the ERM can be seen as a grey-whitish membrane that obscures the visualization of the underlying retinal vasculature and retinal surface. Other associated biomicroscopic findings may include PVD, small intraretinal and preretinal haemorrhages, central macular oedema due to retinal vascular leakage, areas of whitening of the inner retina due to axonoplasmic stasis secondary to ischaemia, foveal ectopia due to macular traction and pseudoholes. A pseudohole is a commonly associated clinical finding and is considered to be the result of the formation of a membrane defect accompanied by the displacement of retinal tissue that occurs during the contraction of the ERM [9]. The Watzke-Allen slit beam test is a useful clinical test that can differentiate between a pseudohole and a true full-thickness macular hole [42]. In cases of a positive Watzke-Allen test, the patient will perceive a "break" in the slit beam. The test is negative in the case of a pseudohole.

Optical coherence tomography (OCT) is the most sophisticated and contemporary imaging modality in the diagnosis of ERMs. In OCT imaging, an ERM is typically demonstrated as a hyperreflective band over the retinal surface, while wrinkling of the retina is easily visualized when present. Associated clinical entities, such as vitreomacular traction, macular oedema, loss of the foveal pit and foveal ectopia due to ERM traction are also readily demonstrated using this imaging technique (Figure 1). Moreover, OCT can easily differentiate between a pseudohole and a true macular hole, and can also serve as a very useful tool in ERM preoperative planning and in postoperative follow-up.

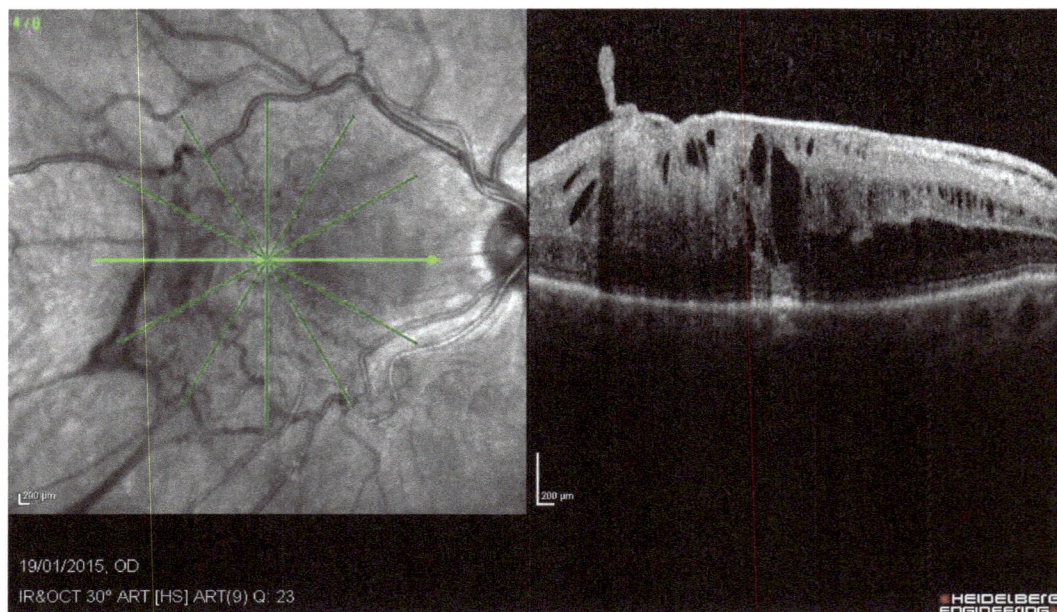

Figure 1. OCT image of an epiretinal membrane. In addition to the apparent thick membrane, the OCT scan reveals considerable macular thickening and cystoid macular oedema. Notice the prominent vascular tortuosity (left) and the obvious edge in the OCT scan of the membrane (right), which may be used for peeling initiation during surgery.

In addition, fluorescein angiography (FA) is another adjuvant diagnostic test for ERM. Despite the fact that it is usually not necessary to establish the diagnosis of an ERM, FA can be helpful in assessing the extent of vascular distortion and detect the presence of vascular leakage and macular oedema. ERM associated vascular leakage, when present, is typically irregular, asymmetric and within the area of the ERM. It is also useful to exclude other lesions that may share common clinical findings with ERMs, such as choroidal neovascularization and other vascular diseases of the retina.

5. Surgical technique and instrumentation

The rationale of the technique for removing the ERM has not changed since 1972, when Machemer introduced this procedure to vitreoretinal surgery. Machemer used a 23g bent needle to remove the epimacular membrane after 17g pars plana vitrectomy. Despite the continuous evolvement and development of surgical instrumentation, the technique today remains practically the same. First, a three-port pars plana vitrectomy is performed. The ERM is then peeled off with appropriate forceps. Dyes are often used to better visualize the membrane. Sometimes, scissors are necessary for the dissection of highly-adhered membranes. Several surgeons proceed to ILM peeling as a next step in order to minimize ERM recurrence. In most cases, the operation finishes without the need for tamponade and mandatory posture.

In the following paragraphs, the steps of the procedure, as well as the necessary equipment and adjuvants are described in more detail.

5.1. Vitrectomy

A three-port pars plana vitrectomy is the first step of the procedure, although there are some reports in the literature regarding direct epiretinal membrane peeling without prior vitrectomy [43-44]. A core vitrectomy is performed, followed by posterior vitreous detachment, if this is not already present. This is done either actively with the vitreous cutter, or passively with a flute needle, starting by elevating the posterior hyaloid membrane at the level of the optic disc. Subsequently, the vitrectomy is completed with the cortex removal.

5.1.1. Microincision Vitrectomy Systems, MIVS

During the past number of years, most surgeons prefer small gauge vitrectomy systems and thus, the procedure is sutureless and atraumatic. The systems that are broadly used for the macula surgery are the 23G and the 25G, while 27G was also recently introduced [45]. The use of either system depends primarily on the surgeon's preference and they do not seem to affect postoperative outcomes [46-49]. However, the wide acceptance of the microincision systems indicates that these outnumber the 20-g system, offering shorter operating times, reduced corneal astigmatism, diminished conjunctival scarring, improved patient comfort and in some cases, earlier visual recovery [50-52]. Although this is true for most vitrectomy applications, it is especially true for macula surgery including ERM peeling.

Small gauge systems are considered to offer better postoperative comfort due to minimal surgical trauma. However, as size goes down, instruments tend to be less stiff, sometimes rendering globe manipulation during surgery difficult. Postoperative leakage from the unsutured entry sites has been correlated to hypotony and endophthalmitis; however, the findings in the literature regarding this are not consistent [48, 50, 53-54]. Moreover, as the small cutter lumen removes smaller vitreous quantities per cut, vitreous removal is relatively slower compared to traditional vitrectomy. Recent advances in vitrectomy systems related to fluidics, cutting rates, instrument design and alloys, have succeeded in compensating for most of these drawbacks and have made microincision vitrectomy systems the preferred platform for most posterior segment surgeons. The introduction of xenon and mercury vapour lights has also helped in overcoming some early problems related to illumination. The bright illumination and low light hazard offered by these light sources, even in very small diameter systems, have helped to broaden the scope of small gauge vitrectomy.

5.1.2. Visualization systems

Extremely clear visualization of the surgical field represents one of the cornerstones of modern retinal microsurgery. Dealing with fine tissues and transparent membranes, and avoiding damage to sensitive structures, requires a very good stereoscopic view. Several systems have been introduced in surgical practice; below, the most commonly used are reviewed.

5.1.2.1. Contact lenses

Plano-concave lenses are placed directly on the cornea for posterior segment view. Their primary advantage is the high-resolution image that the surgeon obtains with their application. However, they have an important disadvantage in the form of their instability during surgery. In order to overcome this limitation, ring systems have been designed for sutureless stabilization on the cornea; at the same time, various ways have been proposed for adjusting them (e. g., on the speculum, at the cannulas etc.). Many surgeons use these lenses either separately or in combination with a non-contact system.

5.1.2.2. Non-contact systems

The first non-contact optical system for visualizing the posterior segment was presented in 1987, which was the binocular indirect ophthalmomicroscope (BIOM, Oculus, Wetzlar, Germany) [55]. It is the most frequently used wide-angle viewing system for retinal surgery. The BIOM, as all other non-contact systems, is based on indirect ophthalmoscopy, which results in an inverted image. An optical system introduced in the microscope's optical pathway is used for image re-inversion, so that the image viewed by the surgeon has normal orientation. An important feature of the BIOM is the variety of lenses that one can choose from and switch between during surgery, as it comes with a 60 deg., 90 deg. and 120 deg. refraction lens. For example, for macular surgery, a 60 deg. macula lens can be placed for the membrane peeling, while at the end of the procedure, the surgeon can switch to a 120 deg. wide field in order to check for breaks at the periphery. In first BIOM generations, the focus and the inversion of the field were manual; however, most recent BIOMs have incorporated a footswitch for focus adjustment and an automated inverter.

Other non-contact systems include the EIBOS (HS, Moeller-Wedel Optical GmbH, Wedel, Germany), the OFFISS (optic fibre free intravitreal surgery system/OFFISS; Topcon Medical

Systems, Oakland, NJ), the OptiFlex (Volk, Mentor, OH), the PWL (PWL; Ocular Instruments, Bellevue, WA) and the Resight 700 (Carl Zeiss Meditec AG, Jena, Germany). Each of them has positive (automatic inverters, adjusted illumination, automatic lens switches, etc.) and negative (adjustable in specific microscopes, unstable coaxiality, etc.) aspects. Eventually, the selection of the particular optical system will depend on the surgeon's experience, comfort and familiarity with the technique and the technology.

5.1.3. Visualization adjuvants

Vital dyes stain the faint epiretinal membranes and thus improve contrast during surgery. Their utilization has considerably facilitated macular surgery and is considered by many surgeons extremely helpful for both ERM and ILM removal [56]. Trypan Blue (TB) is the most frequently used dye and stains mainly the ERM. Brilliant Blue G (BBG) stains both the ILM and ERM and is preferred when ILM removal is also desired. Other dyes such as indocyanine green (ICG) and infracyanine green (IFCG) primarily stain the ILM and we will not discuss their use in this chapter.

The use of trypan blue for ERM staining has been well-studied and is considered an excellent, non-toxic approach for visualizing the membrane [57-59]. It is usually injected under air in order to avoid lens capsule staining; this will hinder the continuation of the operation due to the deprivation of the view of the posterior segment. Alternatively, heavy TB can be used, which does not demand an air-fluid exchange [60]. The TB is left for one- to three-minutes and is then washed away. The epiretinal membrane and other proliferative tissue are stained and their edges show against the unstained background.

Brilliant Blue G mostly stains the ILM, but the ERM is also stained to some degree [61]. It is preferred when dual staining is necessary, for simultaneous removal of ERM and ILM [62]. It is also injected under air and washed away after a few minutes. It is generally reported to be safe although some concerns about retinal toxicity have been raised [59, 63-64].

Another substance that is quite effective in visualizing ERMs is triamcinolone (TA). TA is not a dye; it forms crystals that are deposited through loosely organized collagen matrices, making visible the vitreous body, but also ERMs and the ILM [65].

5.1.4. Forceps and scissors

Fine instruments are imperative for handling fine structures such as the epiretinal membranes and the ILM to lessen possible damage to the underlying retinal tissue. Instrument sizes follow the trend of minimizing the size of the vitrectomy ports. Nowadays, forceps, scrapers, scissors and other adjuncts exist in compatibility with 20g, 23g, 25g and 27g PPV systems.

End-grasping forceps are the most commonly used instruments for ERM peeling. Klaus Eckhardt developed the first fine end-grasping forceps in the 90s; these proved to be very effective and are still preferred today. Later, Charles developed conformal forceps, meaning that they have the same radius of curvature as the retina and avoid grasping of the retinal surface by grasping the nerve fibre layer (NFL) during the procedure. Rarely, in high adherence situations, scissors can be used. Horizontal scissors are preferred because of their safer profile compared to vertical scissors. They can be inserted into the potential space between the membrane and the retina, with both blades more efficiently delaminating the ERM from the subjacent tissue.

When the edge of the membrane is not easily grasped by forceps, a Tano diamond dusted membrane scraper (DDMS) can be used. This tool is coated with inert diamond dust that makes traction easier and offers an atraumatic alternative to finding the edge of the membrane due to its soft silicon tip. The Tano DDMS is for some surgeons an indispensable part of macular surgery. Its use is also suggested for ILM removal. However, attempting to create an edge at the ILM with this tool is strongly discouraged due to the damage it can cause to the subjacent tissue [66].

5.2. Removal technique

Once the vitrectomy is completed, the ERM is inspected for visible edges. Existing edges are visualized much better if dye has been used for ERM staining. Moreover, careful preoperative evaluation using SDOCT can be extremely helpful in this regard by providing information about the 3D configuration of the membrane and the selection of an optimum area for peel initiation. If a pre-existing edge cannot be found, it can be created using a pick or a micro-vitreoretinal (MVR) blade. The edge is then grasped with the forceps, with the one blade on the anterior surface and the other under the membrane, and a circumscribed flap is created. Then, careful and gentle dissection is started from the periphery to the centre of the membrane (outside-in technique), similar to the capsulorhexis in cataract surgery. Alternatively, the membrane is grasped centrally and peeled away from the centre, always in a circumferential pattern (inside-out technique). Some surgeons consider the inside-out technique safer, because the central retina is thicker and stronger, making it easier for the surgeon to find a tissue plane to begin with.

Since both the picking and the grasping of the membrane can cause damage to the subjacent retinal tissue (tears, bleeding, ischaemia), good visualization and controlled manoeuvres are very important at this stage. Directing the tip tangentially to the retinal surface and engaging the membrane from different directions helps to avoid fragmentation of the tissue sheet and inadvertent tearing of the retina [67].

Charles has proposed an alternative approach for minimizing tissue damage, described as "pinch peeling". In this case, the forceps pinch the membrane without creating an "edge" and grasp it with the two blades on the surface of the membrane. Retinal contact is thus avoided and the risk of retinal damage is minimized [68].

5.2.1. ILM peeling

Very often, the ILM is peeled off together with the ERM. This can be monitored during ERM peeling by using a dye that stains both the ERM and the ILM, e. g., Membrane Blue Dual® (DORC, Japan). If this is not achieved, the ILM can be removed at a second step. ILM peeling is impossible without the creation of an opening in the inner limiting membrane. If an edge of the ILM has not been created during ERM manipulation and removal, it can be made using a pick or MVR blade, at a location away from the maculo-papillary bundle, frequently along the temporal horizontal raphe. The fine-end forceps are again used to grasp and elevate the membrane and peeling is again performed in a circular motion, extending towards the vascular arcades. The simultaneous removal of the ILM is imperative for some surgeons, but it is not yet clear whether it affects recurrence rates [69-70] or retinal function [71-73].

5.3. Conclusion of surgery

Following ERM removal, inspection of the peripheral retina follows; if this shows no iatrogenic damage, surgery is completed by trocar removal and sclerotomy closure. If iatrogenic damage is present, breaks in the periphery without subretinal fluid accumulation can be treated by laser retinopexy or cryoretinopexy. The presence of significant amounts of subretinal fluid necessitates internal drainage, retinopexy and gas tamponade.

Although scleral ports in small gauge vitrectomy are designed so that no sutures are necessary, careful inspection of the water tightness of the ports at the conclusion of surgery is mandatory in order to avoid early postoperative hypotony. Gentle massage of the site of scleral incision after trocar removal can improve a relatively leaky incision. Occasionally, the insertion of a small suture may be necessary for a leaky scleral incision.

6. Results and prognosis

6.1. Functional results

In general, visual acuity seems to improve following ERM surgery. More than 50% of patients gain 2 or more logMAR lines and less than 10% end up with lower postoperative VA [74-76]. Preoperative vision is usually 20/63 or worse, but cases with good visual acuity have been reported to benefit from surgery, too [77]. Improvement in vision usually occurs in the first two to three months, but complete recovery may require six to 12 months following surgery. Additionally, cataract extraction is very likely to be needed shortly after ERM peeling, as nuclear sclerosis accelerates after vitrectomy [75, 77-79].

Overall, visual prognosis depends on preoperative vision, the duration of symptoms and the preoperative anatomical status of the fovea and retinal layers [74, 80]. Postoperative BCVA is better in patients with good preoperative VA, but the gain in letters seem to be greater for patients with poorer preoperative VA. This means that patients with low preoperative visual acuity do not enjoy complete recovery after macular membrane removal. Limited restoration of the VA in these patients can be due to chronic traction, which results in permanent retinal vascular incompetence. Subsequent retinal vascular leakage and persistent cystoid macular oedema restrict the restoration of macular function and anatomy.

Metamorphopsia, one of the main reasons for patients deciding to undergo surgery, has not been investigated in a methodical and quantified manner. In the few studies that have studied metamorphopsia, it appears to improve after surgery and can happen as early as the first postoperative month [81-82]. Its preoperative existence affects postoperative visual outcomes, but the duration of preoperative symptoms do not affect the postoperative visual acuity three months after surgery [81].

6.2. Anatomical outcome

Postoperative reduction of the central macular thickness (CMT) has been a consistent finding in most studies [75, 83]. Figure 2 shows the anatomic restoration of the fovea (b) and following the removal of the epimacular membrane (a) in one of our cases, six months postoperatively. Visual recovery, however, is not always correlated with the decrease of retinal thickness. Recent studies have correlated other preoperative and postoperative anatomical features with visual outcomes. OCT represents an invaluable tool for the assessment of these features, primarily by using high definition techniques. Ellipsoid zone (IS/OS) integrity, photoreceptor outer segment (PROS) length and external limiting membrane (ELM) integrity represent some of the anatomical characteristics that appear to play an important role in functional prognosis. Significant changes in ellipsoid integrity (IS/OS) have been correlated with visual outcomes, while postoperative elongation of the PROS have been described in successful cases [84].

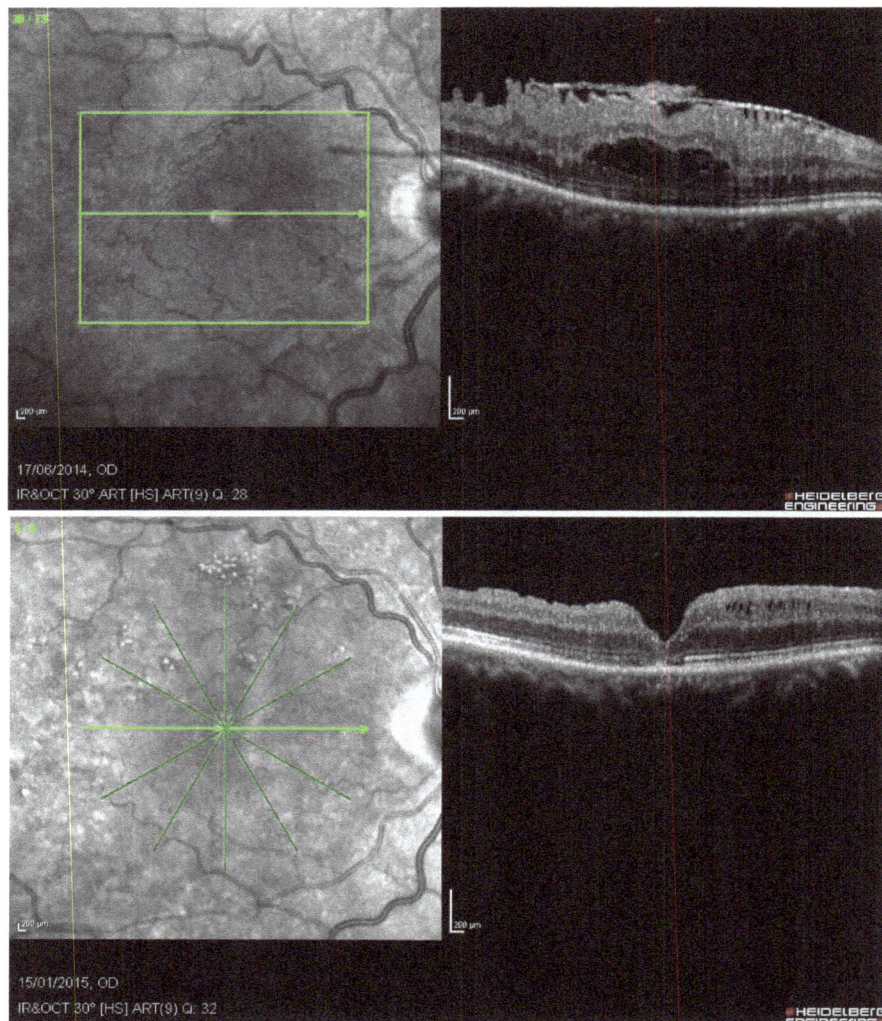

Figure 2. Anatomical restoration after ERM peeling; a) preoperative image of contracted ERM with retinal thickening and cystoid macular oedema; b) six months after surgery the foveal anatomy has greatly improved. Small intraretinal cysts can still be seen along with some changes in the outer retinal layers.

On the other hand, although postoperative visual field loss is known to occur in some cases following ERM surgery, its correlation with anatomical changes in the OCT has not been confirmed by the literature. The effect of surgery on the nerve fibre layer (NFL) and the ganglion cell layer (GCL) are under intense investigation, especially with *"en face"* OCT and other sophisticated techniques. However, the results on whether there is loss of neuronal or glial tissue remain ambiguous, as do reasons for the late deformation of the central retina, often observed following ERM surgery. Based on modern retinal imaging modalities, it is believed that retinal reconstruction continues for months after ERM peeling [85-86].

6.3. Prognosis of different ERM subtypes

Secondary epiretinal membranes have worse prognosis than idiopathic membranes [69]. Limited visual recovery, as well as higher recurrence rates, is reported. Diabetic membranes are difficult to manage, as they are accompanied by severe retinal damage that can lead to serious complications including haemorrhage, detachment and re-proliferation of the connective tissue [87]. Postoperative ERMs (including ERMs developed after vitrectomy for retinal detachment, but also after laser or cryo-retinopexy) have limited visual recovery, especially when the macula is detached [88]. Finally, inflammatory membranes illustrate variable results, depending mostly on the effect of the subjacent inflammation on the retinal function [89].

7. Complications

Epiretinal membrane removal is generally a safe procedure. Intraoperative complications involve retinal breaks, retinal haemorrhage, retinal whitening and retinal surface damage. Postoperative complications include cataract formation, rhegmatogenous retinal detachment (RRD), cystoid macular oedema, endophthalmitis and the recurrence of fibrotic tissue.

A common intraoperative complication is the creation of iatrogenic retinal breaks. These occur during vitrectomy; thus, careful examination of the periphery with indentation at the conclusion of surgery is crucial for their early/prompt diagnosis. Their treatment is straightforward, that is, through the application of intraoperative laser retinopexy or cryopexy. However, a break can also occur at the posterior pole (due to pinching or during the dissection of a high-adherent membrane) and in this case, laser treatment may be hazardous to the fovea and should be performed with caution.

Haemorrhage at the site of pinching or grasping or at the area where the membrane detaches from a retinal vessel is also common. In this case, recovery is usually short and uneventful. More extensive bleeding may occur less often when a vessel is damaged during the dissection and can be controlled by increasing intraocular pressure or intraoperative cautery.

Retinal whitening is the result of ischaemia that usually resolves intraoperatively; nevertheless, sometimes it may persist for an extended period of time. Membrane manipulation can also cause surface tissue damage, which may or may not be symptomatic. Symptoms involve primarily visual field defects and one should differentiate if these are due to tissue deficits or ischaemia. In the first case, direct damage may be the result of pinching or gripping of the membrane; additionally, indirect damage to the inner retina can occur if ILM peeling had been part of the surgical procedure.

The most frequent postoperative complication of ERM surgery is the progression of nuclear sclerosis of the crystalline lens. Most often, visual acuity improves during the first six to nine months, but then slowly decreases as the cataract develops. The majority of phakic patients undergo cataract extraction within two years in order to maximize the benefits of the initial operation. For this reason, some surgeons prefer a combined operation of phacoemulsification, ERM peeling and IOL implantation [74-76, 90].

Rhegmatogenous retinal detachment is another important postoperative event. The cause in this case is usually a peripheral break caused by traction or incarceration of vitreous in the sclerotomies and demands surgical treatment.

Recurrence of ERMs may be seen in up to 5% of eyes with idiopathic membranes. Younger individuals, patients with a prior history of retinal detachment and patients with a prior history of uveitis tend to have a higher recurrence rate, which in some studies have been up to 12% [71]. Remarkably, recurrence is reported to be higher by many studies when ILM is left intact [69, 91].

Endophthalmitis is quite rare after standard 20g vitrectomy (0.02 to 0.14%) [92]. For transconjuctival sutureless vitrectomy (TSV) and especially when using the 25g system, higher rates have been reported (0.04 to 1.55%) [92]. Nevertheless, this finding has not been conclusively confirmed in the literature; thus, the question regarding the increased risk of infection after TSV is yet to be clarified [93-97].

8. Surgery vs. observation

Despite the favourable results of surgery for the treatment of ERM, debate remains regarding a preferable treatment strategy. Decision for surgery and selection of the proper method depends on the surgeon's preference and on the patients' characteristics. Nevertheless, it is highly significant to perform meticulous patient selection for each method in order to achieve better outcomes with regard to patients' overall visual ability and quality of life.

As discussed above, interventional studies indicate that early surgical removal can relieve disturbing symptoms and stabilize vision, which may worsen later [74-77, 81-82]. This is in contrast with the fact that ERMs do not always progress and may be stable during follow-up without any intervention [35, 98]. Moreover, there are possible side effects to surgery and the improvement in visual acuity is greater in patients with preoperative lower visual acuity.

In the paragraphs that follow, we will attempt to review data from the literature concerning surgery timing and patient selection.

Epidemiological population-based studies suggest that a large percentage of cases diagnosed with ERM may remain stable during follow-up. These studies agree that the disease is non-progressive in a significant percentage of cases and also that regression may be observed without any intervention. In the Blue Mountains eye study, 28.6% of cases experienced progression, 38.8% of eyes remained stable and 25.7% of cases regressed in a five-year follow-up period [35]. In a prospective cohort study of 1932 patients undergoing cataract surgery, it was reported that 43% of patients progressed postoperatively after one month had passed during a 36-month follow-up, 32.4% of patients remained stable and 24.6% of patients regressed [98]. According to these results, similar percentages of patients with cellophane maculopathy and patients with preretinal fibrosis progressed; additionally, the regression rates in both groups were similar: 26% of cellophane reflex cases and 18% of preretinal fibrosis cases regressed spontaneously without surgical intervention. Of the 14 cases of preretinal fibrosis regression, five cases had complete regression, while the rest had partial ERM regression. In the Blue Mountains study, regression rates were similar in the cellophane macular reflex (CMR) group and in the preretinal macular fibrosis (PMF) group (25.7% and 25.8%, respectively). Regarding progression, 16.1% of participants with PMF at baseline and 32.8% of patients with CMR at baseline progressed, including 17 eyes in which CMR progressed to PMF (9.3%). There was no significant association between the ocular and systemic risk factors detected for predicting the progression of preretinal macular fibrosis during the five-year follow-up [35]. It appears that according to these prospective cohort studies, progression of ERM affected about a third of patients; furthermore, a small amount of patients regressed completely. The differences in percentages among studies can be attributed to the different criteria selected for progression and regression, as well as to the different study populations.

Based on these data, a follow-up period prior to making a decision for surgery was imposed in most cases, depending on the amount of visual disturbance upon diagnosis.

Regarding visual acuity, in the Blue Mountains study, the authors demonstrated that the level of mean visual acuity was only slightly affected by incident preretinal macular fibrosis and was unaffected by incident cellophane macular reflex. The average reduction of visual acuity after five years in the worst eyes was 5.7 letters (CI, 5.3 to 6.1) in subjects without incident epiretinal membranes, 7.4 letters (CI, 4.7 to 10.1) in eyes with incident preretinal macular fibrosis and 2.8 letters (CI, 1.6 to 4.0) in eyes with incident cellophane macular reflex. Corresponding mean differences in visual acuity between the baseline and a five-year examination were not statistically significant [35]. Thus, surgery was not promptly needed with regard to visual acuity, since the progression of vision loss, if any, was very slow. When surgery is undertaken in cases with significantly impaired visual acuity, it provides improvement more frequently and to a greater extent than in eyes with better preoperative visual acuity [79].

On the other hand, eyes with lower preoperative visual acuity tend to have lower final visual acuity, whereas the final visual prognosis is better for eyes with better preoperative visual acuity [79, 99]. Studies using spectral domain optical coherence tomography have shown that visual disturbance induced by ERM is associated with intraretinal changes, including the disruption of photoreceptor integrity. These findings suggest that the damage resulting from ERMs is partially irreversible, regardless of surgical management. Consequently, from this point of view, an early intervention prior to the induction of permanent damage seems more rational.

In order to make the decision for undergoing surgery, it is important to evaluate the prognosis of surgery in each case. Preoperative evaluation with time-domain OCT (TDOCT) and spectral-domain OCT (SDOCT) has given us the ability to assess morphologic features that correspond to intraretinal tissue damage and its association with preoperative visual symptoms, and to evaluate the potential for improvement [81, 100-103]. According to clinical studies with TDOCT and SDOCT, the preoperative disruption of the photoreceptors' inner and outer segment junction (ellipsoid zone, IS/OS) is one of the main prognostic factors. Suh et al. and Falkner-Radler et al. compared TDOCT in ERM patients pre- and post- vitrectomy and found that eyes experiencing disruption of the ellipsoid zone had significantly lower postoperative best corrected visual acuity (BCVA) and lower BCVA differences when comparing pre- and post-surgery conditions, compared to those without preoperative OCT disruption [81, 100]. The latter study additionally confirmed the predictive value of ellipsoid zone integrity for postoperative functional outcomes with SDOCT [100]. Inoue et al. and Kim et al. prospectively allocated their patients based on preoperative ellipsoid zone integrity in groups of intact versus disrupted and found that the intact ellipsoid zone cohort had better final visual acuity and better improvement in visual acuity. The predictive role of the preoperative central foveal thickness, the presence of a macular pseudohole or the presence of retinal cysts was not confirmed in these studies [101-103].

Other factors that may predict visual outcome and affect decisions regarding surgery are the presence of any other macular co-morbidity such as age-related maculopathy. The length of the photoreceptor outer segment and the thickness of the inner retinal layer are also correlated with visual function, and might therefore be useful in predicting surgical outcomes [103]. Additionally, as mentioned earlier, the presence and severity of metamorphopsia has also been correlated with final visual outcomes [81-82].

9. Conclusion

Vitrectomy and membrane peeling is currently the preferred surgical treatment option for eyes with ERM. However, no consensus has been established concerning an optimal time for surgery. Early intervention may prevent the evolvement of non-reversible damage to the outer retina; however, ERM progression concerns only a small percentage of patients. Follow-up with SDOCT and clinical examination for recording visual acuity and metamorphopsia is imposed in early cases prior to decision-making. Moreover, in more advanced stages, the application of SDOCT for assessing retinal integrity and predicting postoperative outcomes is necessary in order to predict possible functional gain following surgery.

Author details

Miltiadis K. Tsilimbaris*, Chrysanthi Tsika, George Kontadakis and Athanassios Giarmoukakis

*Address all correspondence to: tsilimb@med.uoc.gr

University of Crete, Medical School, Department of Ophthalmology, Crete, Greece

References

[1] Iwanoff A. Beiträge zur normalen und pathologischen Anatomie des Auges. Graefes Arch Clin Exp Ophthalmol. 1865; 11: 135-70.

[2] Sidd RJ, Fine SL, Owens SL, Patz A. Idiopathic preretinal gliosis. Am J Ophthalmol. 1982;94:44-8.

[3] Sheard RM, Sethi C, Gregor Z. Acute macular pucker. Ophthalmology. 2003; 110: 1178-1184.

[4] Rivellese M, George A, Sulkes D, Reichel E, Puliafito C. Optical coherence tomography after laser photocoagulation for clinically significant macular edema. Ophthalmic Surg Lasers. 2000; 31: 192-197.

[5] Hassenstein A, Bialasiewicz AA, Richard G. Optical coherence tomography in uveitis patients. Am J Ophthalmol. 2000; 130: 669-670

[6] Uemura A, Ideta H, Nagasaki H, Morita H, Ito k. Macular pucker after retinal detachment surgery. Ophthalmic Surg. 1992;23:116-9.

[7] Appiah AP, Hirose T. Secondary causes of premacular fibrosis. Ophthalmology. 1989;96:389-92.

[8] Meyers SM, Gutman FA, Kaye LD, Rothner AD. Retinal changes associated with neurofibromatosis 2.Trans Am Ophthalmol Soc 1995; 93: 245-52.

[9] Gass JDM. Macular dysfunction caused by epiretinal membrane contraction. In: Stereoscopic Atlas of Macular Diseases: Diagnosis and Treatment. Vol. 2, 4th ed. St Louis, Mo: Mosby; 1997:938-50.

[10] Mitchell P, Smith W, Chey T, Wang JJ, Chang A. Prevalence and associations of epiretinal membranes. The Blue Mountains Eye Study, Australia. Ophthalmology 1997; 104: 1033-40.

[11] Pearlstone AD. The incidence of idiopathic preretinal macular gliosis. Ann Ophthalmol. 1985;17:378-80.

[12] Roth AM, Foos RY. Surface wrinkling retinopathy in eyes enucleated at autopsy. Trans Am Acad Ophthalmol Otolaryngol. 1971;75(5):1047-58.

[13] Duan XR1, Liang YB, Friedman DS, Sun LP, Wei WB, Wang JJ, Wang GL, Liu W, Tao QS, Wang NL, Wong TY. Prevalence and associations of epiretinal membranes in a rural Chinese adult population: the Handan Eye Study. Invest Ophthalmol Vis Sci. 2009; 50(5):2018-23.

[14] Clarkson JG, Green WR, Massof D. A histopathologic review of 168 cases of preretinal membrane. Am J Ophthalmol. 1977;84(1):1-17.

[15] Uemura A, Ideta H, Nagasaki et al. Macular pucker after retinal detachment surgery. Ophthalmic Surg. 1992;23:116-9.

[16] Lobes LA Jr., Burton TC. The incidence of macular pucker after retinal detachment surgery. Am J Ophthalmol. 1978;85:72-7.

[17] Michels RG, Wilkinson CP, Rice TA. Retinal detachment. St Louis: CV Mosby; 1990:1096-8.

[18] Smiddy WE, Maguire AM, Green et al. Idiopathic epiretinal membranes. Ultrastructural characteristics and clinicopathologic correlation. Ophthalmology 1989; 96:811-821.

[19] Yamashita H, Hori S, Masuda K. Population and proportion of component cells in preretinal membranes. Jpn J Ophthalmol 1986; 30:269-281.

[20] Kampik A, Kenyon KR, Michels RG, Green WR, de la Cruz ZC. Epiretinal and vitreous membranes. Comparative study of 56 cases. Arch Ophthalmol 1981; 99:1445-1454.

[21] Hirokawa H, Jalkh AE, Takahashi et al. Role of the vitreous in idiopathic preretinal macular fibrosis. Am J Ophthalmol. 1986;101:166-9.

[22] Hikichi T, Takahashi M, Trempe CL, Schepens CL. Relationship between premacular cortical vitreous defects and idiopathic premacular fibrosis. Retina. 1995;15(5):413-6.

[23] Heilskov TW, Massicotte SJ, Folk JC. Epiretinal macular membranes in eyes with attached posterior cortical vitreous. Retina. 1996;16:279-84.

[24] Kampik A. Pathology of epiretinal membrane, idiopathic macular hole, and vitreomacular traction syndrome. Retina. 2012; 32(2):194-8

[25] Cherfan GM, Smiddy WE, Michels et al. Clinicopathologic correlation of pigmented epiretinal membranes. Am J Ophthalmol. 1988;106:536-45.

[26] Snead DR, James S, Snead MP. Pathological changes in the vitreoretinal junction 1: epiretinal membrane formation. Eye (Lond). 2008 Oct;22(10):1310-7.

[27] Harada C, Mitamura Y, Harada T. The role of cytokines and trophic factors in epiretinal membranes: involvement of signal transduction in glial cells. Prog Retin Eye Res. 2006; 25(2):149-64.

[28] Harada T, Harada C, Mitamura Y, Akazawa C, Ohtsuka K, Ohno S, Takeuchi S, Wada K. Neurotrophic factor receptors in epiretinal membranes after human diabetic retinopathy. Diabetes Care. 2002 Jun;25(6):1060-5.

[29] Chen YS, Hackett SF, Schoenfeld CL, Vinores MA, Vinores SA, Campochiaro PA. Localisation of vascular endothelial growth factor and its receptors to cells of vascular and avascular epiretinal membranes. Br J Ophthalmol. 1997;81(10):919-26.

[30] Minchiotti S, Stampachiacchiere B, Micera A, Lambiase A, Ripandelli G, Billi B, Bonini S. Human idiopathic epiretinal membranes express NGF and NGF receptors. Retina. 2008; 28(4):628-37.

[31] Iannetti L, Accorinti M, Malagola R, Bozzoni-Pantaleoni F, Da Dalt S, Nicoletti F, Gradini R, Traficante A, Campanella M, Pivetti-Pezzi P. Role of the intravitreal growth factors in the pathogenesis of idiopathic epiretinal membrane. Invest Ophthalmol Vis Sci. 2011; 52(8):5786-9.

[32] Mandelcorn E, Khan Y, Javorska L, Cohen J, Howarth D, Mandelcorn M. Idiopathic epiretinal membranes: cell type, growth factor expression, and fluorescein angiographic and retinal photographic correlations. Can J Ophthalmol. 2003 ;38(6):457-63.

[33] Joshi M, Agrawal S, Christoforidis JB. Inflammatory mechanisms of idiopathic epiretinal membrane formation. Mediators Inflamm. 2013;2013:192582.

[34] Mandal N, Kofod M, Vorum H, Villumsen J, Eriksen J, Heegaard S, Prause JU, Ahuja S, Honoré B, la Cour M. Proteomic analysis of human vitreous associated with idiopathic epiretinal membrane. Acta Ophthalmol. 2013; 91(4):333-4.

[35] Fraser-Bell S, Guzowski M, Rochtchina et al. Five-Year Cumulative Incidence and Progression of Epiretinal Membranes The Blue Mountains Eye Study. Ophthalmology 2003;110:34-40.

[36] Hayashi K, Hayashi H. Influence of phacoemulsification surgery on progression of idiopathic epiretinal membrane. Eye. 2009; 23(4):774-9.

[37] Charlap RS, Yagoda AD, Debbi S, Bodine SR, Walsh JB, Henkind P. Idiopathic preretinal macular gliosis: a retrospective study of 200 patients. Ann Ophthalmol. 1992; 24(10):381-5.

[38] Wiznia RA. Natural history of idiopathic preretinal macular fibrosis. Ann Ophthalmol. 1982; 14:876-878.

[39] Wise GN. Clinical features of idiopathic preretinal macular fibrosis. Am J Ophthalmol. 1975; 79:349-357.

[40] Messner KH. Spontaneous separation of preretinal macular fibrosis. Am J Ophthalmol. 1977; 83:9-11.

[41] Tadayoni R, Paques M, Massin P, Mouki-Benani S, Mikol J, Gaudric A. Dissociated optic nerve fiber layer appearance of the fundus after idiopathic epiretinal membrane removal. Ophthalmology 2001;108:2279-83.

[42] Tanner V, Williamson TH. Watzke-Allen slit beam test in macular holes confirmed by optical coherence tomography. Arch Ophthalmol. 2000;118(8):1059-63.

[43] Sawa M, Saito Y, Hayashi A, Kusaka S, Ohji M, Tano Y. Assessment of nuclear sclerosis after nonvitrectomizing vitreous surgery. Am J Ophthalmol. 2001;132(3):356-62.

[44] Longo A, Avitabile T, Bonfiglio V, Toro MD, Russo A, Viti F, Nicolai M, Saitta A, Giovannini A, Mariotti C. Transconjunctival nonvitrectomizing vitreous surgery versus 25-gauge vitrectomy in patients with epiretinal membrane: A Prospective Randomized Study. Retina 2014 [In Press].

[45] Oshima Y, Wakabayashi T, Sato T, Ohji M, Tano Y. A 27-gauge instrument system for transconjunctival sutureless microincision vitrectomy surgery. Ophthalmology 2010;117:93-102 e102.

[46] El Sanharawi M, Lecuen N, Barale PO, Bonnel S, Basli E, Borderie V, Laroche L, Monin C. 25-, 23-, and 20-gauge vitrectomy in epiretinal membrane surgery: a comparative study of 553 cases. Graefes Arch Clin Exp Ophthalmol. 2011;249(12):1811-9.

[47] Grosso A, Charrier L, Lovato E, Panico C, Mariotti C, Dapavo G, Chiuminatto R, Siliquini R, Gianino MM. Twenty-five-gauge vitrectomy versus 23-gauge vitrectomy in the management of macular diseases: a comparative analysis through a Health Technology Assessment model. Int Ophthalmol. 2014;34:217-223.

[48] Haas A, Seidel G, Steinbrugger I, Maier R, Gasser-Steiner V, Wedrich A, Weger M. Twenty-three-gauge and 20-gauge vitrectomy in epiretinal membrane surgery. Retina 2010;30:112-116.

[49] Kusuhara S, Ooto S, Kimura D, Itoi K, Mukuno H, Miyamoto N, Akimoto M, Kuriyama S, Takagi H. Outcomes of 23- and 25-gauge transconjunctival sutureless vitrectomies for idiopathic macular holes. Br J Ophthalmol. 2008;92(9):1261-4.

[50] Rizzo S, Genovesi-Ebert F, Murri S, Belting C, Vento A, Cresti F, Manca ML. 25-gauge, sutureless vitrectomy and standard 20-gauge pars plana vitrectomy in idiopathic epiretinal membrane surgery: a comparative pilot study. Graefes Arch Clin Exp Ophthalmol. 2006;244(4):472-9.

[51] Goncu T, Gurelik G, Hasanreisoglu B. Comparison of efficacy and safety between transconjunctival 23-gauge and conventional 20-gauge vitrectomy systems in macular surgery. Korean J Ophthalmol. 2012;26(5):339-46.

[52] Galway G, Drury B, Cronin BG, Bourke RD. A comparison of induced astigmatism in 20- vs 25-gauge vitrectomy procedures. Eye 2010;24:315-317.

[53] Valmaggia C. Pars plana vitrectomy with 25-gauge instruments in the treatment of idiopathic epiretinal membranes. Klin Monbl Augenheilkd. 2007;224:292-296.

[54] Thompson JT. Advantages and limitations of small gauge vitrectomy. Surv Ophthalmol. 2011;56:162-172.

[55] Spitznas M. A binocular indirect ophthalmomicroscope (BIOM) for non-contact wide-angle vitreous surgery. Graefes Arch Clin Exp Ophthalmol. 1987;225:13-15.

[56] Hernandez F, Alpizar-Alvarez N, Wu L. Chromovitrectomy: an update. Journal of ophthalmic & vision research 2014;9:251-259.

[57] Kwok AK, Lai TY, Li WW, Yew DT, Wong VW. Trypan blue- and indocyanine green-assisted epiretinal membrane surgery: clinical and histopathological studies. Eye. 2004;18:882-888.

[58] Feron EJ, Veckeneer M, Parys-Van Ginderdeuren R, Van Lommel A, Melles GR, Stalmans P. Trypan blue staining of epiretinal membranes in proliferative vitreoretinopathy. Arch Ophthalmol. 2002;120:141-144.

[59] Creuzot-Garcher C, Acar N, Passemard M, Bidot S, Bron A, Bretillon L. Functional and structural effect of intravitreal indocyanine green, triamcinolone acetonide, trypan blue, and brilliant blue g on rat retina. Retina. 2010;30:1294-1301.

[60] Lesnik Oberstein SY, Mura M, Tan SH, de Smet MD. Heavy trypan blue staining of epiretinal membranes: an alternative to infracyanine green. Br J Ophthalmol. 2007;91:955-957.

[61] Totan Y, Guler E, Dervisogullari MS. Brilliant Blue G assisted epiretinal membrane surgery. Sci Rep. 2014;4:3956.

[62] Shimada H, Nakashizuka H, Hattori T, Mori R, Mizutani Y, Yuzawa M. Double staining with brilliant blue G and double peeling for epiretinal membranes. Ophthalmology 2009;116:1370-1376.

[63] Penha FM, Pons M, Costa Ede et al. Effect of vital dyes on retinal pigmented epithelial cell viability and apoptosis: implications for chromovitrectomy. Ophthalmologica. 2013;230 Suppl 2:41-50.

[64] Penha FM, Pons M, Costa EF, Barros NM, Rodrigues EB, Cardoso EB, Dib E, Maia M, Marin-Castaño ME, Farah ME. Retinal pigmented epithelial cells cytotoxicity and apoptosis through activation of the mitochondrial intrinsic pathway: role of indocyanine green, brilliant blue and implications for chromovitrectomy. PloS one 2013;8:e64094.

[65] Konstantinidis L, Berguiga M, Beknazar E, Wolfensberger TJ. Anatomic and functional outcome after 23-gauge vitrectomy, peeling, and intravitreal triamcinolone for idiopathic macular epiretinal membrane. Retina 2009;29:1119-1127.

[66] Kuhn F, Mester V, Berta A. The Tano Diamond Dusted Membrane Scraper: indications and contraindications. Acta Ophthalmol Scand. 1998;76:754-755.

[67] Bopp, S. 2005.Is There Room for Improvement in Pucker Surgery? In: Kirchhof, B. & Wong, D. ed Vitreo-retinal Surgery, Essentials in Ophthalmology. Berlin Heidelberg. Springer, pp: 37-65.

[68] Charles S. Techniques and tools for dissection of epiretinal membranes. Graefes Arch Clin Exp Ophthalmol. 2003;241:347-352.

[69] Kang KT, Kim KS, Kim YC. Surgical results of idiopathic and secondary epiretinal membrane. Int Ophthalmol. 2014;34:1227-1232.

[70] Oh HN, Lee JE, Kim HW, Yun IH. Clinical outcomes of double staining and additional ILM peeling during ERM surgery. Korean J Ophthalmol. 2013;27:256-260.

[71] Sandali O, El Sanharawi M, Basli E, Bonnel S, Lecuen N, Barale PO, Borderie V, Laroche L, Monin C. Epiretinal membrane recurrence: incidence, characteristics, evolution, and preventive and risk factors. Retina. 2013;33:2032-2038.

[72] Kwok A, Lai TY, Yuen KS. Epiretinal membrane surgery with or without internal limiting membrane peeling. Clin Experiment Ophthalmol. 2005;33:379-385.

[73] Abdelkader E, Lois N. Internal limiting membrane peeling in vitreo-retinal surgery. Surv Ophthalmol. 2008;53:368-396.

[74] Moisseiev E, Davidovitch Z, Kinori M, Loewenstein A, Moisseiev J, Barak A. Vitrectomy for idiopathic epiretinal membrane in elderly patients: surgical outcomes and visual prognosis. Curr Eye Res. 2012;37:50-54.

[75] Lee PY, Cheng KC, Wu WC. Anatomic and functional outcome after surgical removal of idiopathic macular epiretinal membrane. Kaohsiung J Med Sci. 2011;27:268-275.

[76] Chuang L-H, Wang N-K, Chen et al. Comparison of visual outcomes after epiretinal membrane surgery. Taiwan J Ophthalmol. 2012;2:56-59.

[77] Thompson JT. Vitrectomy for epiretinal membranes with good visual acuity. Trans Am Ophthalmol Soc. 2004;102:97-103; discussion 103-105.

[78] Lee JW, Kim IT. Outcomes of idiopathic macular epiretinal membrane removal with and without internal limiting membrane peeling: a comparative study. Jpn J Ophthalmol. 2010;54:129-134.

[79] Song SJ, Kuriyan AE, Smiddy WE. Results and Prognostic Factors for Visual Improvement after Pars Plana Vitrectomy for Idiopathic Epiretinal Membrane. Retina 2015 [In press].

[80] Benhamou N, Massin P, Spolaore R, Paques M, Gaudric A. Surgical management of epiretinal membrane in young patients. Am J Ophthalmol. 2002;133:358-364.

[81] Falkner-Radler CI, Glittenberg C, Hagen S, Benesch T, Binder S. Spectral-domain optical coherence tomography for monitoring epiretinal membrane surgery. Ophthalmology. 2010;117:798-805.

[82] Kinoshita T, Imaizumi H, Okushiba U, Miyamoto H, Ogino T, Mitamura Y. Time course of changes in metamorphopsia, visual acuity, and OCT parameters after successful epiretinal membrane surgery. IOVS. 2012;53:3592-3597.

[83] Kim J, Rhee KM, Woo SJ, Yu YS, Chung H, Park KH. Long-term temporal changes of macular thickness and visual outcome after vitrectomy for idiopathic epiretinal membrane. Am J Ophthalmol. 2010;150:701-709.

[84] Hashimoto Y, Saito W, Saito M, Hirooka K, Fujiya A, Yoshizawa C, Noda K, Ishida S. Retinal outer layer thickness increases after vitrectomy for epiretinal membrane, and visual improvement positively correlates with photoreceptor outer segment length. Graefes Arch Clin Exp Ophthalmol. 2014;252:219-226.

[85] Pichi F, Lembo A, Morara M, Veronese C, Alkabes M, Nucci P, Ciardella AP. Early and late inner retinal changes after inner limiting membrane peeling. Int Ophthalmol. 2014;34:437-446.

[86] Kumagai K, Ogino N, Furukawa M, Hangai M, Kazama S, Nishigaki S, Larson E. Retinal thickness after vitrectomy and internal limiting membrane peeling for macular hole and epiretinal membrane. Clin Ophthalmol. 2012;6:679-688.

[87] Hsu YR, Yang CM, Yeh PT. Clinical and histological features of epiretinal membrane after diabetic vitrectomy. Graefes Arch Clin Exp Ophthalmol. 2014;252:401-410.

[88] Martinez-Castillo V, Boixadera A, Distefano L, Zapata M, Garcia-Arumi J. Epiretinal membrane after pars plana vitrectomy for primary pseudophakic or aphakic rhegmatogenous retinal detachment: incidence and outcomes. Retina. 2012;32:1350-1355.

[89] Tanawade RG, Tsierkezou L, Bindra MS, Patton NA, Jones NP. Visual Outcomes of Pars Plana Vitrectomy with Epiretinal Membrane Peel in Patients with Uveitis. Retina. 2014 [In Press].

[90] Yiu G, Marra KV, Wagley S, Krishnan S, Sandhu H, Kovacs K, Kuperwaser M, Arroyo JG. Surgical outcomes after epiretinal membrane peeling combined with cataract surgery. Br J Ophthalmol. 2013;97:1197-1201.

[91] Pournaras CJ, Emarah A, Petropoulos IK. Idiopathic macular epiretinal membrane surgery and ILM peeling: anatomical and functional outcomes. Semin Ophthalmol. 2011;26:42-46.

[92] Dave VP, Pathengay A, Schwartz SG, Flynn HW Jr. Endophthalmitis following pars plana vitrectomy: a literature review of incidence, causative organisms, and treatment outcomes. Clin Ophthalmol. 2014;8:2183-2188.

[93] Hu AY, Bourges JL, Shah SP, Gupta A, Gonzales CR, Oliver SC, Schwartz SD. Endophthalmitis after pars plana vitrectomy a 20- and 25-gauge comparison. Ophthalmology. 2009;116:1360-1365.

[94] Scott IU, Flynn HW Jr, Acar N, Dev S, Shaikh S, Mittra RA, Arevalo JF, Kychenthal A, Kunselman A. Incidence of endophthalmitis after 20-gauge vs 23-gauge vs 25-gauge pars plana vitrectomy. Graefes Arch Clin Exp Ophthalmol. 2011;249:377-380.

[95] Govetto A, Virgili G, Menchini F, Lanzetta P, Menchini U. A systematic review of endophthalmitis after microincisional versus 20-gauge vitrectomy. Ophthalmology. 2013;120:2286-2291.

[96] Scott IU, Flynn HW Jr, Dev S, Shaikh S, Mittra RA, Arevalo JF, Kychenthal A, Acar N. Endophthalmitis after 25-gauge and 20-gauge pars plana vitrectomy: incidence and outcomes. Retina. 2008;28:138-142.

[97] Eifrig CW, Scott IU, Flynn HW, Jr., Smiddy WE, Newton J. Endophthalmitis after pars plana vitrectomy: Incidence, causative organisms, and visual acuity outcomes. Am J Ophthalmol. 2004;138:799-802

[98] Fong CS, Mitchell P, Rochtchina E, Hong T, de Loryn T, Wang JJ. Incidence and progression of epiretinal membranes in eyes after cataract surgery. Am J Ophthalmol. 2013 Aug;156(2):312-318.

[99] Pesin SR, Olk RJ, Grand MG, Boniuk I, Arribas NP, Thomas MA, Williams DF, Burgess D. Vitrectomy for premacular fibroplasia. Prognostic factors, long-term follow-up, and time course of visual improvement. Ophthalmology. 1991 Jul;98(7):1109-14.

[100] Suh MH, Seo JM, Park et al. Associations between macular findings by optical coherence tomography and visual outcomes after epiretinal membrane removal. Am J Ophthalmol 2009;147:473-80.

[101] Inoue M, Morita S, Watanabe et al. Inner segment/outer segment junction assessed by spectral-domain optical coherence tomography in patients with idiopathic epiretinal membrane. Am J Ophthalmol 2010;150:834-9.

[102] Inoue M, Morita S, Watanabe et al. Preoperative inner segment/outer segment junction in spectral-domain optical coherence tomography as a prognostic factor in epiretinal membrane surgery. Retina 2011;31:1366-72.

[103] Kim HJ, Kang JW, Chung H, Kim HC. Correlation of foveal photoreceptor integrity with visual outcome in idiopathic epiretinal membrane. Curr Eye Res. 2014 Jun;39(6): 626-33.

4

Eye Removal — Current Indications and Technical Tips

César Hita-Antón, Lourdes Jordano-Luna and Rosario Díez-Villalba

Abstract

The removal of the eyeball with or without other orbital tissues is always a complicated decision to take and nearly always involves the beginning of a new and intense doctor-patient relationship. The loss of the globe results in the loss of binocular vision and depth perception, thus the patient is limited when applying for certain jobs or handling delicate or dangerous materials. They may also be prohibited to drive in some countries o may have to do so with special care where permitted. The psychological impact on the patients′ life may be even greater as it may be perceived as a severe facial disfiguration. Some patients may prefer to stay at home and their social life may be deeply affected. Since facial and eye appearance is essential for normal human relations and interaction, prosthetic eyes or orbits should imitate the eye, in most cases, or the whole orbit-eyelids-eye complex, which is less frequent.

Keywords: enucleation, evisceration, exenteration, orbital implant

1. Introduction

The need to remove an eye or other orbital contents is always difficult to digest for a patient. Many of them will experience the five stages of grief described by the Swiss psychiatrist Elisabeth Kübler-Ross in her 1969 book [1] *On Death and Dying*, inspired by her work with terminally ill patients. Older patients may think that these kinds of surgeries, especially exenteration, are not worth it. Younger patients are usually very worried about the cosmetic result rather than the difficulty of the surgery and the postoperative period. The ophthalmologist will need a good dose of empathy and psychology skills to explain to the patient that the planned surgery is the only and best option. The oculoplastic surgeon must be ready to hear that some patients will wish to ask for a second opinion. This may annoy the doctor in charge of the patient, but despite of this, it is advisable to help the patient look for a second opinion with other colleagues. When dealing with these kinds of patients, it is crucial to take your time to explain with detail the surgical technique, the time the patient is expected to stay in the hospital, the need for frequent bandage changes in the hospital clinic, the possible complications of the socket, and a long recovery period before a prosthesis can be fitted in.

Evisceration, enucleation, and exenteration are the three main surgical options. Evisceration is the removal of the contents of the globe while leaving the sclera and extraocular muscles intact. Enucleation is the removal of the eye from the orbit while preserving all the other orbital structures, and exenteration is the removal of the globe as well as the soft tissues of the orbit (connective tissue, fat, and muscles).

There is evidence that Egyptians and Sumerians used artificial eyes to decorate their mummies and their statues, respectively; however, there is no evidence to suggest that they used them for medical purposes in living people. Clay models resembling eyes were used in the Roman Empire around 500 BC to cover phthisical eyes. It was not until the 16th century that enucleation surgeries were reported in the medical literature. In 1583, George Bartisch first described the extirpation of an eye. In 1817, Bear introduced evisceration in an eye with an expulsive hemorrhage when performing an iridectomy for an acute glaucoma [2].

It was in 1874 when Noyes reported the routine evisceration of the ocular contents when there was severe intraocular infection [3]. Later, in 1884, Mules reported for the first time the use of an orbital glass sphere implant in an eviscerated cavity, this becoming the bedrock of volume loss restoration and improving dramatically cosmetic results of this surgery [2,4]. In 1887, Frost inserted a crystal ball orbital implant inside Tenon's capsule after an enucleation procedure [5].

Since then, advances in surgical techniques, anesthesia, new implants, and wrapping materials and prosthetics over the past decade have greatly improved surgical outcomes and patient satisfaction. Today, most patients have good cosmetic results following the removal of and eye. However, even an exquisite surgical technique cannot prevent complications in the immediate and long-term follow-up of these sockets, making these patients challenging for the Oculoplastic Surgeon.

The decision to remove an eye must be individualized to each patient. Advantages and disadvantages exist among the different surgical techniques and implant materials.

2. Surgical indications

2.1. Enucleation

The most common indications are intraocular malignancy, blind painful eyes, penetrating trauma, very bad ocular cosmesis or phthisical eyes, and prevention of sympathetic ophthalmia (SO).

A significant decrease in the number of enucleations was observed between 1975 and 1995. This was primarily caused by a decrease in the number of glaucoma-related enucleations [6]. Evisceration, unlike enucleation, disrupts the integrity of the globe's barriers, which could trigger an autoimmune reaction (SO) in the contralateral eye. Although some authors believe that SO continues to be an important disadvantage, evisceration has gained popularity in the past few decades because of superior functional and cosmetic results compared to enucleation. Levine et al. [7] concluded that the risk of SO following evisceration is extremely low.

Choroidal melanoma in adults and retinoblastoma in children are the most common intraocular malignancies. In some cases of malignancy diathermy, chemotherapy and radiation may be an alternative to more disfiguring surgeries.

2.2. Evisceration

1. Penetrating trauma: one of the most common indications of evisceration in cases when sclera is largely intact. Classically, it was thought that surgery should be performed within 14 days of injury. In cases with extensive disruption of the globe's tissues, the removal of all uveal tissue is difficult via an evisceration; therefore, enucleation may be a better option [6].

2. Blind eyes: removal of a blind eye is generally the last possibility. We attempt to control pain with a retrobulbar injection of alcohol or chlorpromazine. When the patient refers corneal discomfort, some eyes may benefit from conjunctival flaps [8]. Nowadays evisceration is widely preferred in Europe because of its advantages in blind eyes, such as better cosmetic results and shorter postoperative recovery time [9].

3. Endophthalmitis: many surgeons prefer evisceration for endophthalmitis because of the low risk of bacterial retroocular space invasion. Others suggest that enucleation should be performed when there is no certainty that the sclera may be involved [10]

2.3. Exenteration

Orbital content removal is reserved for the treatment of potentially life-threatening malignances arising from the eye, eyelid, orbit, paranasal sinuses, and periocular skin. Secondary orbital spread from eyelid, intraocular, and conjunctival malignant tumors was the most frequent indication of exenteration, followed by primary orbital malignant tumors. Other indications have included sclerosing inflammatory pseudotumors and invasive fungal disease of the orbit [11-13].

3. Surgical techniques

3.1. Enucleation surgical technique

1. It is absolutely mandatory to ensure we will remove the correct eye. Sometimes it is obvious which eye should be enucleated, like in a severely traumatized eye, but in other cases, the eye can be morphologically perfect and doubts can arise. This can be the case of a choroidal melanoma. We strongly recommend to read the patients notes and ask the patient to identify the eye that should be removed. Once sure, the eye should be marked with pen with an arrow or letters on the side of the forehead of that eye. We also like to

dilate the eye with tropicamide [14]. This marks the side to operate on and allows the surgeon to check the tumor inside the globe in the operating room.

2. Once in the operating room, we ask the patient to identify calling out his name and surname and age. We ask again which eye is the one to be removed and to signal it for us with his hand before he lies on the operating table.

3. Although we are aware some surgeons prefer intravenous sedation and local anesthesia, it is of our preference and of our patients to undergo general anesthesia. Even in cases of general anesthesia, some surgeons also inject local anesthesia so as to obtain local vasoconstriction, which will aid the surgeon making the surgery "cleaner" and faster. Two percent lidocaine with 1:100,000 epinephrine can be used for superficial injection like in the subconjunctival space. Retrobulbar anesthesia is made with a combination of 2% lidocaine and 1:100,000 epinephrine mixed 1:1 with 75% bupivacaine.

4. Intravenous antibiotic is usually used 30 min prior to surgery in the presurgery preparation area.

5. We prep and drape in the standard fashion using povidone iodine for the skin and conjunctiva. We like to cover the other eye, but some may prefer to let the other eye uncovered and closed.

6. We use a lid speculum, taking care to protect the field from eyelashes. If eyelashes enter the field, these can be cut or stuck to the eyelid with an adhesive skin closure.

7. Using Westcott scissors or dissection scissors, perform a 360° limbal peritomy trying to leave on the limbus no more than 1 mm of conjunctiva. Remember to be as careful as possible. The conjunctiva, once closed at the end of the surgery, will be the first defensive layer of the anopthalmic socket (Figure 1).

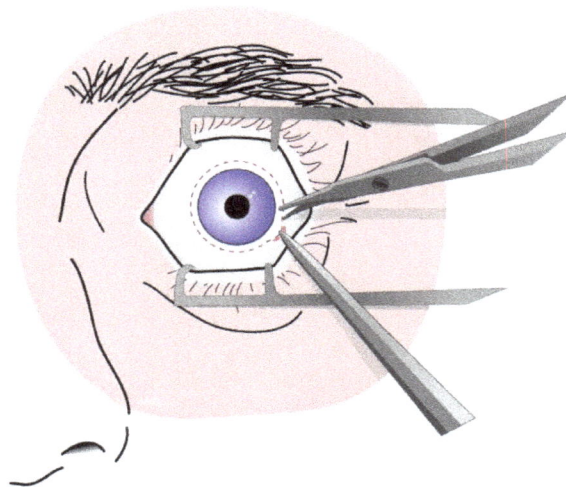

Figure 1. 360° limbal peritomy

8. Blunt dissect Tenon's capsule from the globe. Introduce your dissection scissors beneath the conjunctiva and Tenon in the limbus in any of the four quadrants limited by the four

rectus muscles and smoothly direct your dissection posteriorly and around the globe until you feel you are close to the optic nerve. Repeat this maneuver in the other three quadrants (Figure 2).

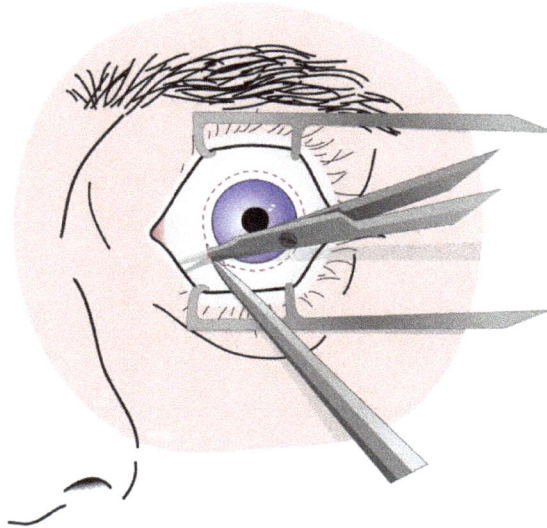

Figure 2. Blunt dissection of Tenon's capsule

9. Localize each rectus muscle with one or two muscle hooks. Ensure you isolate the insertion of the muscle. If this is not visible, some Tenon tissue may be present. Remove it with blunt forceps, pulling it away from the muscle insertion (Figure 3).

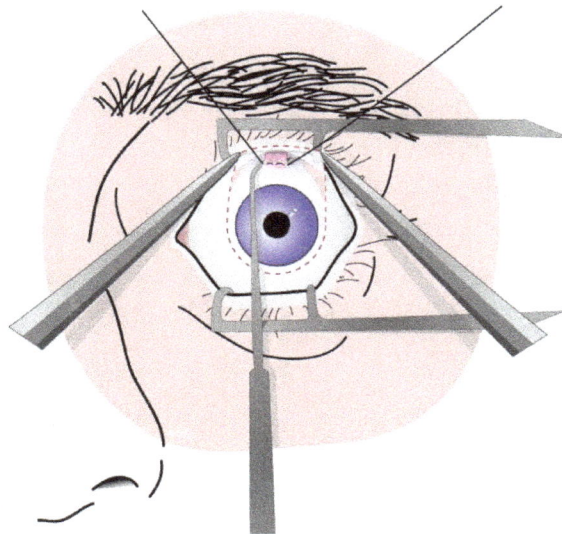

Figure 3. Muscle insertion isolation

10. Pass a 5/0 absorbable suture in a whiplock fashion on either side of the muscles insertion. Cauterize with a monopolar (Colorado needle) or bipolar cautery to avoid bleeding and

then cut the insertion of the muscle with a scissor leaving 1 or 2 mm of insertion on the globe (this stump will be useful in the future to pull the eye out of the orbit). Clamp the sutures for the four rectus muscles away from the surgical field with bulldog clamps or hemostats. The muscles will "spread" away from the globe (Figures 3-5).

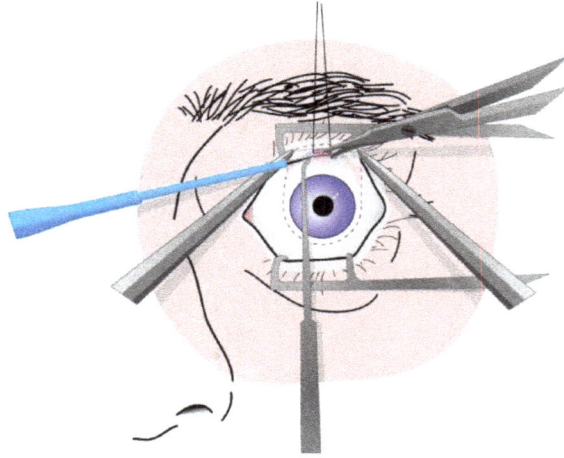

Figure 4. Muscle insertion is cut

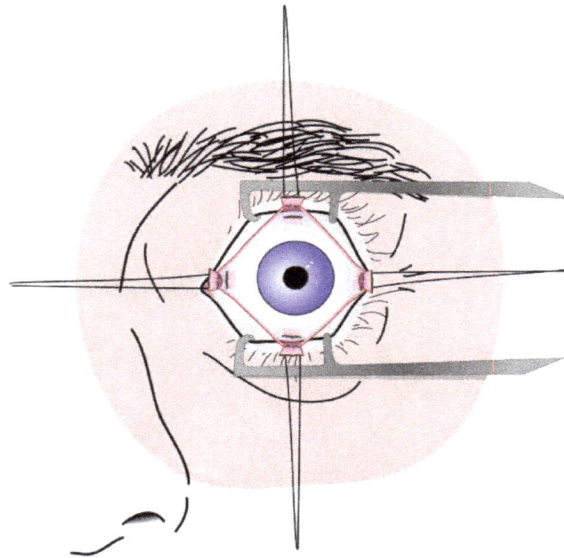

Figure 5. Four rectus muscles are isolated

11. Isolate the inferior oblique muscle in the inferotemporal quadrant with a muscle hook sweeping it from posterior to anterior toward where the inferior rectus was located. As with the rectus muscles, cauterize and cut. Some surgeons like to reinsert the inferior oblique muscle in the orbital implant. In our experience, it is not necessary to achieve a correct implant motility (Figure 6).

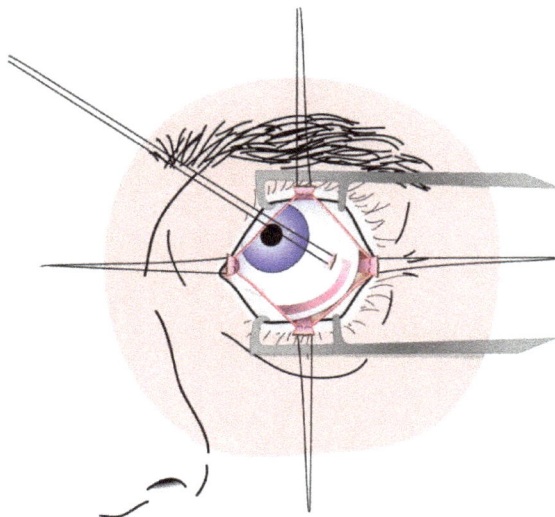

Figure 6. Inferior oblique exposure

12. Isolate the superior oblique muscle in the superonasal quadrant by sweeping the muscle hook from anterior to posterior toward the insertion of the superior rectus muscle. Cauterize, cut, and leave untagged.

13. Pass a 4/0 silk suture through the insertion of the two horizontal rectus muscles or the four of them. This will help to pull the globe during the removal.

14. Place a hemostat around the optic nerve. This will prevent the ophthalmic artery from bleeding. Place a large curved hemostat behind the globe; thus, you can safely cut the optic nerve with scissors without danger for the integrity of the globe. When you cut the nerve, you will find it harder than you would expect. To get as much optic nerve stump as possible, try to direct the scissors posteriorly while pulling the globe out of the orbit with your traction sutures (Figures 7 and 8).

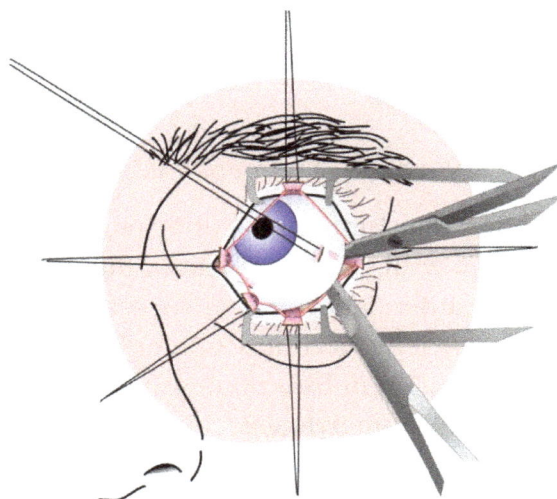

Figure 7. Hemostat placed on optic nerve which is cut with scissors

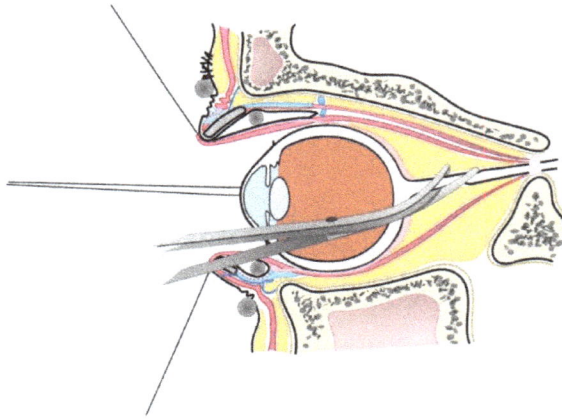

Figure 8. Sagital view of the orbita showing the optic nerve being cut

15. Once the nerve is cut and you pull with your silk sutures, you may feel something is retaining the globe in the orbit. It is usually small segments of retained Tenon's capsule. Cut this Tenon's tissue with care as it may contain small vessels that may bleed. We recommend you cut this tissue as close to the globe as possible in order to avoid inadvertent injury to other tissues like muscles or orbital fat (Figure 9).

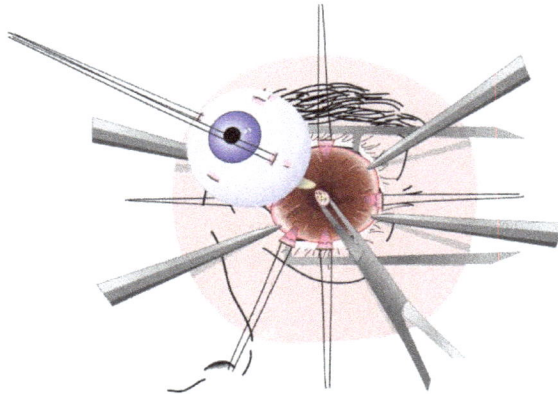

Figure 9. Globe removed from the orbit. Optic nerve stump compressed by hemostat

16. Place the globe in an auxiliary table and prepare it to send to the pathologist.

17. Release the hemostat around the stump of the optic nerve. Apply pressure in the socket and coagulate the optic nerve with the monopolar or bipolar cautery if there is generous bleeding. Avoid excessive cauterization in the socket as it may predispose to future complications of the cavity such as its contraction or implant displacement. Sometimes gentle pressure with gauze soaked in thrombin, saline, or hydrogen peroxide for a few minutes is enough to stop small hemorrhages.

18. Once the socket is ready, the next step is to introduce the orbital implant. The size of which should have been chosen depending of the axial length of the eye or the fellow eye if the removed eye was in phthisis.

19. Nonporous implants should be implanted, wrapped in a mesh or donor sclera; porous implants can be implanted, wrapped or unwrapped.

20. Prior to insertion of the implant, it is immersed in an antibiotic solution (500 mg of cefazolin in 500 ml of saline). Then a Vicryl mesh or sclera is placed around de implant. If you use a mesh, twist the excess mesh in the posterior pole of the implant, tie a knot with 4/0 polyglactin suture, and cut the remaining material. If you use donor sclera, suture it around the implant with 5/0 silk.

21. The implant is then introduced within Tenon's capsule in the orbit. Some surgeons use a Carter sphere introducer or similar plunger-like mechanisms. We use our hands. It is of crucial importance in order to avoid future problems to place the implant as posterior as possible. This is in the intraconal space, leaving part of the posterior pole of the implant uncovered by Tenon's capsule. Sometimes Tenon's tissue is dragged as you introduce the implant. We recommend that the surgical assistant retracts Tenon's anteriorly so as to avoid its displacement with nontoothed forceps while placing the implant.

22. Once correctly positioned in the orbit, we press the implant deep in the orbit with a finger to make sure it is correctly fitted. Make sure that Tenon's layer is not trapped under the implant and that it covers the implant needing no excessive traction with nontoothed forceps. If any doubt of good positioning or implant size should arise, removal of the implant is always a good option.

23. Secure the rectus muscles on the anterior surface of the implant or on the wrapping material. We like to suture first the horizontal rectus muscles. Avoid overlapping of the muscles. Some authors recommend a 5-to-10mm distance between them. We believe that placing them next to each other helps preventing implant extrusion. In the same way, suture both vertical rectus muscles adjacent to the horizontal muscles, creating a "muscle barrier." You may want to suture the inferior oblique muscle just inferior to the lateral rectus muscle (Figures 10 and 11).

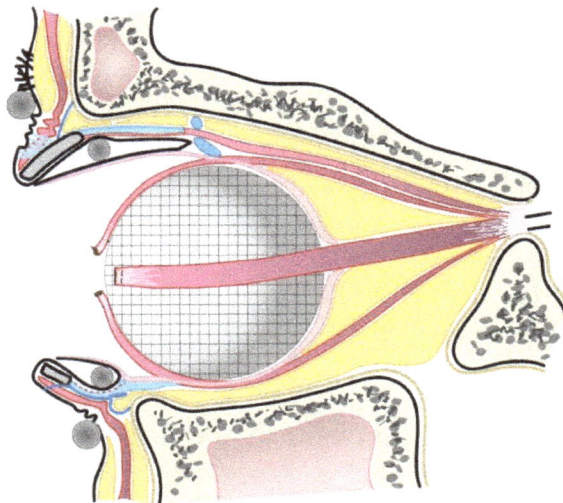

Figure 10. Sagital view of the orbit showing four rectus muscles sutured to the implant

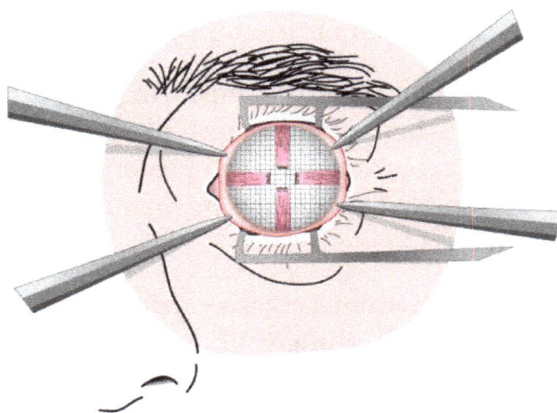

Figure 11. Frontal view of the orbit showing four rectus muscles sutured to the implant

24. Meticulous closure of Tenon's capsule is very important. We recommend interrupted buried 5/0 absorbable (polyglactyn) sutures, but some may prefer a running suture. It is extremely important to avoid tension when closing Tenon's layer (Figure 12).

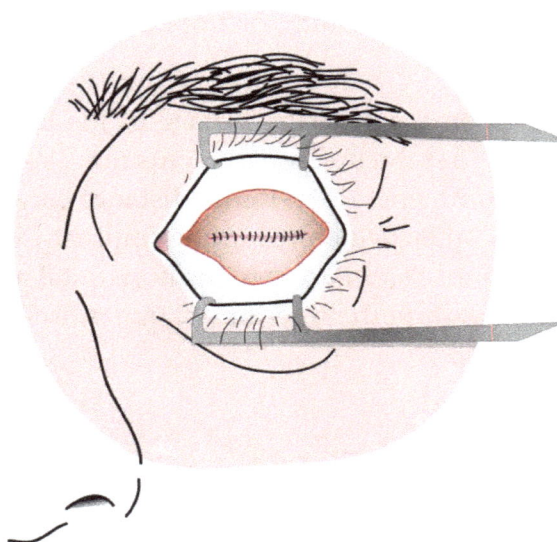

Figure 12. Tenon's capsule sutured beneath conjunctiva

25. A running 6/0 absorbable suture is used to close the conjunctiva, once again, avoiding not too close tissue under tension. Nerad [14] recommends local anesthetic injection into the retrobulbar space for postoperative pain relief (Figure 13). We prefer intravenous analgesia.

26. Abundant antibiotic and steroid ointment should be placed in the socket, and finally an acrylic conformer should be placed. Some surgeons perform a temporal tarsorrhaphy to maintain the conformer in place for 1 or 2 weeks.

27. Tight application of eye patches will finish our surgery.

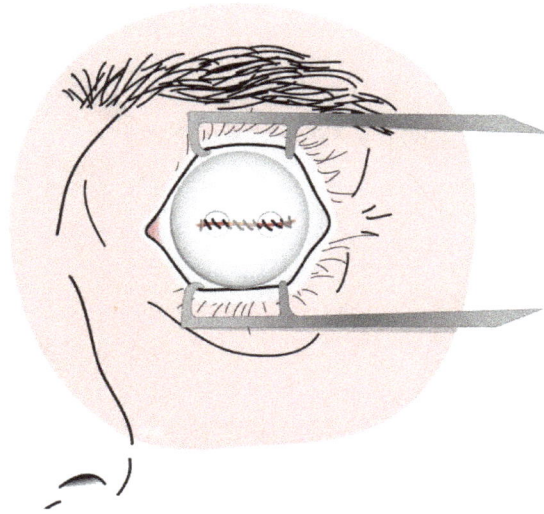

Figure 13. Conjunctiva sutured under an acrylic conformer

3.2. Evisceration surgical technique

1. See enucleation surgical technique (Figure 1).

2. Undermine the conjunctiva by approximately 5 mm, 360°.

3. Blunt dissect Tenon's capsule from the globe. Introduce your dissection scissors beneath the conjunctiva and Tenon's layer in the limbus in any of the four quadrants limited by the four rectus muscles and smoothly direct your dissection posteriorly and around the globe until you feel you are close to the optic nerve. Repeat this maneuver in the other three quadrants (Figure 2).

4. Localize each rectus muscle with one or two muscle hooks. Ensure you isolate the insertion of the muscle. If this is not visible, some Tenon tissue may be present, remove it with blunt forceps pulling it away from the muscles insertion (Figure 3).

5. Pass a 5/0 absorbable suture in a whiplock fashion on either side of the muscles insertion. Clamp the sutures for the four rectus muscles away from the surgical field with bulldog clamps or hemostats (Figure 14).

6. Incise full thickness of the cornea at the limbus with a blade (numbers 11 and 15; Phaco Keratome). Note that aqueous humor will exit the anterior chamber. Complete a 360° keratectomy with Westcott scissors and toothed forceps (Figure 14).

7. Once the cornea is removed, use an evisceration spoon to dissect the sclera from the choroid. If complete dissection is possible, remove the intraocular contents en bloc. It is common to find active bleeding from the central retinal artery and other perforant arteries that branch from long anterior ciliary arteries. We recommend to use suction and a monopolar or bipolar cautery to stop the bleeding. Should the intraocular contents break while dissecting the choroid from the sclera, we recommend to remove them with a suction device in order to minimize the exposure of the content of the eye to the socket, thus reducing the low risk of sympathetic ophthalmia (Figure 15).

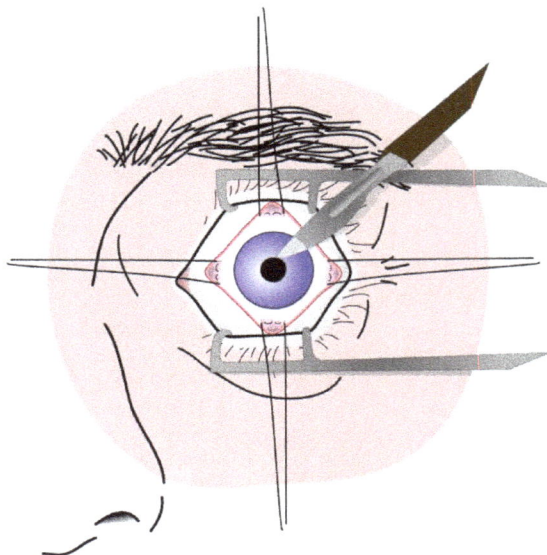

Figure 14. Keratectomy is started with number 15 or number 11 blades

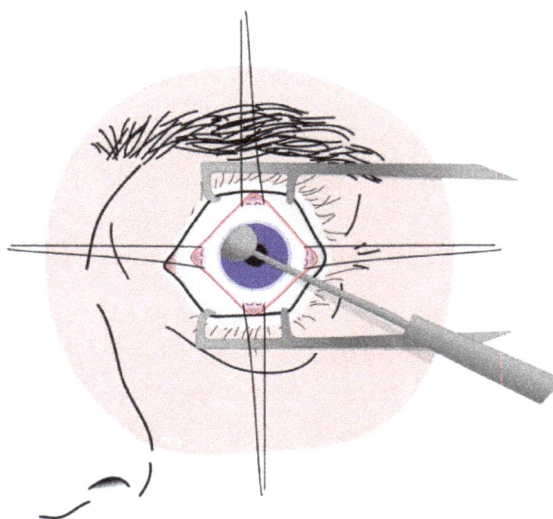

Figure 15. Choroid is dissected from sclera

8.   Wipe the internal scleral surface with cotton-tipped applicators soaked in absolute alcohol and remove retained uveal tissue with gauze.

9.   Upon this point of the surgery, there are different options to prepare the sclera to accommodate the orbital implant. Some authors prefer to make 10-15 mm radial scleral incisions in the four oblique quadrants, avoiding the insertions of the rectus muscles [13]. Others prefer a complete posterior sclerotomy, transecting the sclera from the superior nasal and inferior temporal limbus to the optic nerve. Sclera is then trimmed from the optic nerve in a circular fashion. We prefer the four-petal technique described by Sales-Sanz and Sanz-Lopez [15]: four sclerotomies are performed from the limbus, between the rectus muscle insertions, to the optic nerve with Stevens scissors. The optic nerve is cut at its insertion

point in the posterior sclera. The four sclerotomies reach one another to form four separate scleral petals, each containing one rectus muscle insertion. This last option allows in our experience an easier insertion of the orbital implant in the intraconal space and secondarily makes complete cover of the implant very simple (Figure 16).

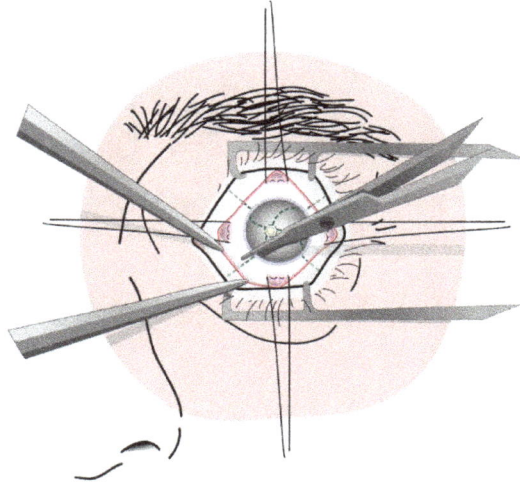

Figure 16. Four sclerotomies performed with scissors

10. 9. Gently pull the four petals out of the socket so the implant can be placed as deep as possible using a Carter sphere introducer or your fingers. The further the implant enters the orbit, the easier it will be to bring the four petals anterior to the implant. Because the petals are independent from each other and from the optic nerve, the sclera can cover any size of implant without tension. The vertical petals are sutured to each other in front of the implant using a continuous 5/0 absorbable suture. The horizontal petals are sutured in the same way over the vertical petals. Make sure that sutures are tied with no tension (Figures 17-20).

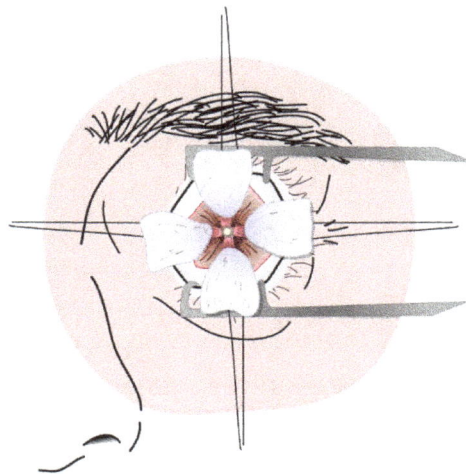

Figure 17. Four petals stretched wide appart

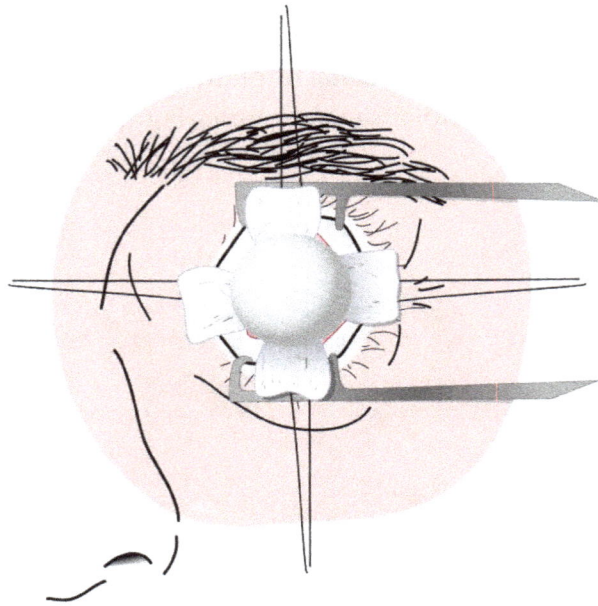

Figure 18. Impant placed between petals pressed deep inside the orbit

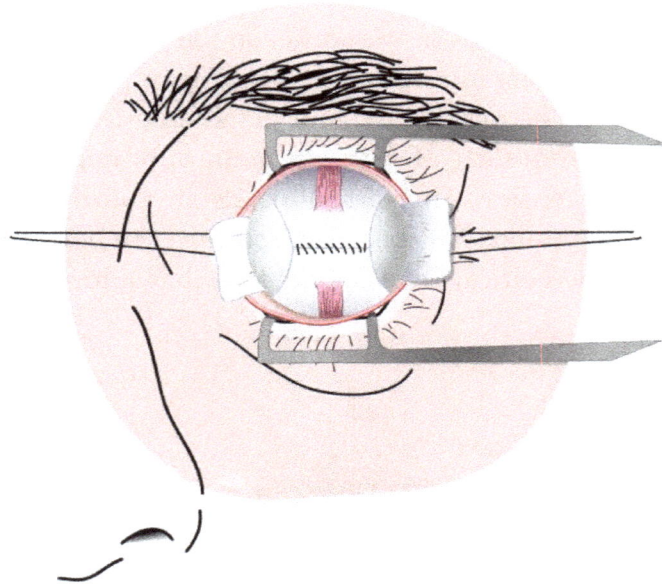

Figure 19. Implant wrapped with sclera from the upper and lower petals with muscles attached

11. Meticulous closure of Tenon's capsule is very important. We recommend interrupted buried 5/0 absorbable (polyglactyn) sutures; again, some may prefer running sutures. It is extremely important to avoid tension when closing Tenon's layer (Figure 12).

12. A running 6/0 absorbable suture is used to close the conjunctiva, once again avoiding to close tissue under tension (Figure 13).

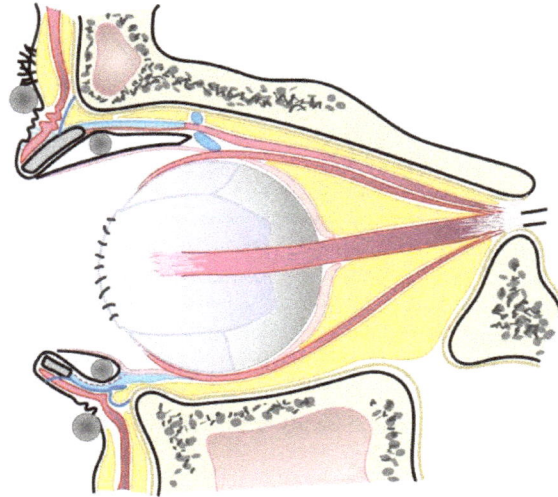

Figure 20. Sagital view of orbit showing correct wrapping of implant with four petals of sclera

13. Abundant antibiotic and steroid ointment should be placed in the socket, and finally an acrylic conformer should be placed. Some surgeons perform a temporal tarsorrhaphy to maintain the conformer in place for 1 or 2 weeks.

14. Tight application of eye patches will finish our surgery.

3.3. Exenteration technique

Technically, orbital exenteration has several variations, each with its own indications.

3.4. Total exenteration

1. General anesthesia is advisable. Local anesthesia is useful to achieve good hemostasis in the eyelid and periorbital tissues. Retrobulbar or intraorbital anesthesias are forbidden when tumors or infections are present.

2. Intravenous antibiotic is usually used 30 min prior to surgery in the presurgery preparation area.

3. 4/0 silk sutures (two per eyelid) are placed on the eyelid border to provide traction. We recommend long bits with the needle as traction later on in the surgery may tear the tarsal and skin tissues.

4. With a scalpel blade (number 11 or 15) or with an electrocautery, incise the skin in an elliptical fashion trying to follow the inner surface of the orbital rim (Figure 21).

5. Dissect under the skin until you reach the periorbita with scissors or with the electrocautery. We strongly recommend to have a bayonet bipolar cautery forceps and a suction device before entering the subperiosteal space (Figure 22).

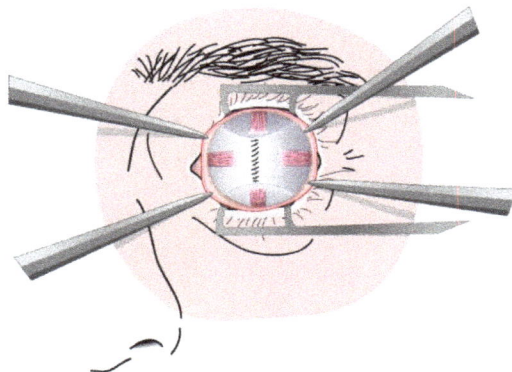

Figure 21. Frontal view of implant wrapped in scleral petals with attached rectus muscles

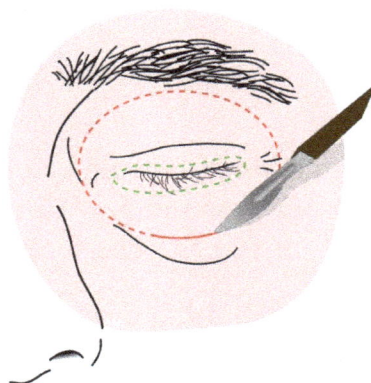

Figure 22. Skin incisión with number 11 or number 15 blades following the inner surface of the orbital rim

6. Once the periorbita is reached, incise it with a scalpel blade, a monopolar cautery, or a Freer periosteal elevator. Sometimes it is difficult to elevate the periorbital periostium as it is firmly stuck to the underlying bone, especially in the frontal bone and the frontal process of the maxillary bone (Figure 23).

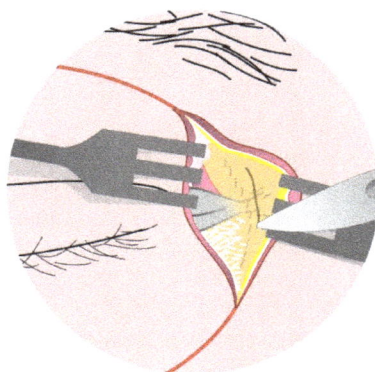

Figure 23. Detail of the periorbita being incised. Note ROOF being rejected temporally and lateral tarsal ligament being rejected nasally

7. Once elevated the periorbital periostium, continue elevating the orbital periosteum. Care should be taken where the periosteum is more tightly adhered to the bone: anterior and posterior lacrimal crests, insertion of the inferior oblique muscle, trochlea, lateral orbital tubercule, and superior and inferior orbital fissures (Figure 24).

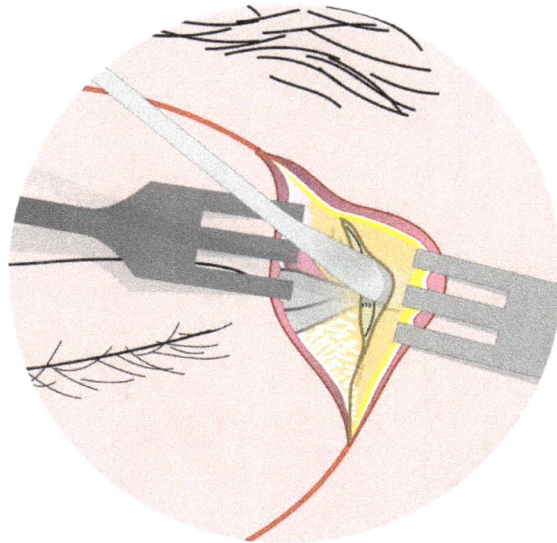

Figure 24. Freer periostal elevator dissecting periorbita

8. Periosteum should elevate easily with the help of the Freer periosteal elevator and malleable retractors. At some point, periosteum can tear, do not panic, and carefully try to dissect it from the opposite point of the tear. The nasolacrimal duct will be exposed once the periosteum is elevated. If possible, obliterate it with fat or muscle to decrease the risk of fistula formation.

9. Continue posterior dissection of the periosteum. At this point, you should remember the orbital anatomy, a squared based pyramid. This means you will need to use your traction sutures on the eyelids and help yourself with one or two small malleable retractors to displace the orbital contents in order to increase the visibility of the orbital walls.

10. Important landmarks to take into account and to avoid damaging are as follows: in the medial wall—supratrochlear and anterior and posterior neurovascular bundles; in the roof—supraorbital neurovascular bundle; in the lateral wall—zygomaticofacial and zygomaticotemporal neurovascular bundles; and in the floor of the orbit—the infraorbital canal. When you come across these structures, bipolar cautery should be applied. Some authors prefer to clip them (Figures 25 and 26).

11. It is also important to remember that the medial wall and the floor of the orbit are easy to break because the bones at those points are thin, especially in the lacrimal fossa and in the ethmoid bone's lamina papyracea.

12. When dissection progresses in the inferolateral portion of the orbit, we will encounter the infraorbital fissure that is rich in vessels. It should be thoroughly electrocauterized.

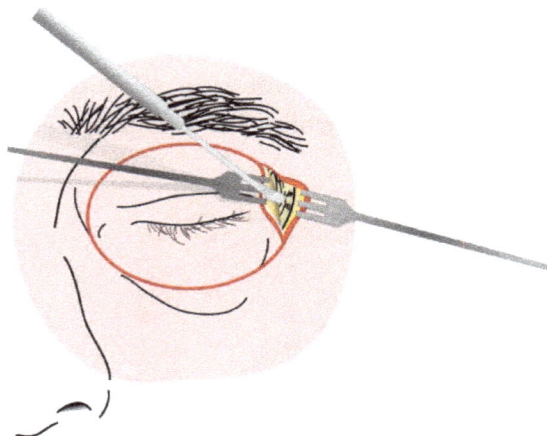

Figure 25. Dissection is carried on deep back towards the orbital apex

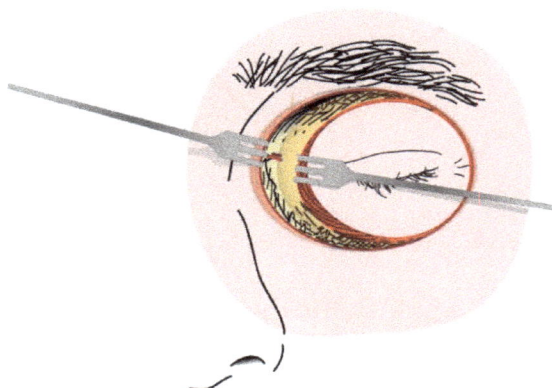

Figure 26. Avoid damaging important vessels such as the Anterior Ethmoidal Artery

13. Continue the dissection until the apex is reached. Carefully cauterize the superior orbital fissure and the posterior orbital tissues, including the optic nerve. We recommend to be patient and slowly cauterize and cut in small bits to avoid bleeding that may be difficult to control and may frighten the surgeon (Figure 27).

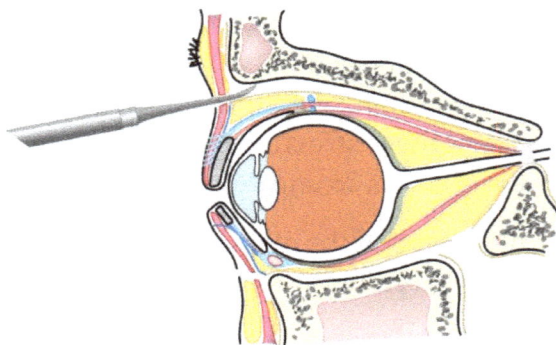

Figure 27. Sagital view of Freer periostal elevator dissecting the periorbita posteriorly

14. Pull the silk traction sutures and place the orbital content in an independent table where it will be prepared to be sent to the pathologist.

15. The orbit with the bare bones may be left to granulate, gauzes with antibiotic should be placed, and the orbit should be pressure patched. Some authors will consider covering the bone with a split-thickness skin graft [11,14,16] from the thigh or a tissue flap, generally from the temporalis muscle (Figures 28 and 29).

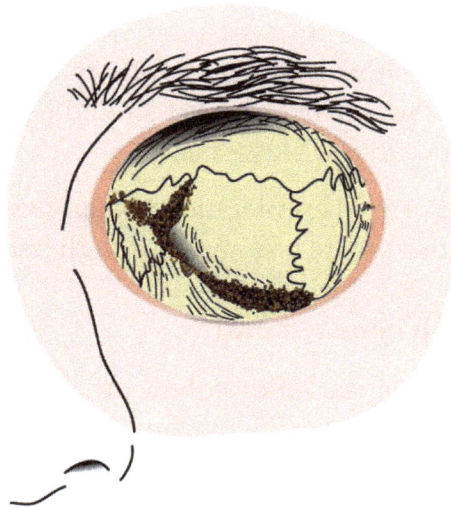

Figure 28. Frontal view of the exenterated orbit showing bone landmarks and hemostasis of the orbital apex

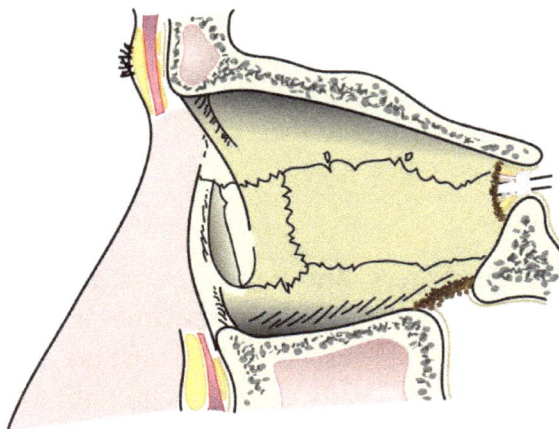

Figure 29. Medial view of the exenterated orbit showing bone landmarks and hemostasis of the orbital apex

3.5. Eyelid-sparing exenteration

We prefer this procedure when the disease does not affect the eyelid because the skin and orbicularis muscle can be used as "primers" to initiate the cavity's granulation and epithelialization. The difference with the previously described technique is that the skin incisions are placed 2 mm above the lash line and are joined at the medial and lateral canthus. Dissection is carried out in the preseptal plane or in the preorbicularis plane. We prefer the preseptal plane; it is easy to follow and allows a good blood supply to the future granulation tissues.

In conclusion, with this procedure, we partly cover the orbital bones, and we add a vascular supply to our skin flap, reducing the time the socket needs to granulate.

3.6. Subtotal exenteration

It may be performed when the disease involves anterior orbit or conjunctiva as in conjunctival melanoma or sebaceous cell carcinoma without evidence of deep orbital invasion. It spares orbital tissues from the deep orbit; thus, the socket should heal earlier, but orbital prosthesis fixation can be complicated since there is less space.

The technique is similar to that of total exenteration but subperiosteal dissection is not carried out as far posteriorly. Orbital tissues are cut, and thorough hemostasia is performed.

3.7. Extended exenteration with bone removal

Unfortunately, high-grade malignancies or osteolytic processes will require total exenteration and the removal of the bones of the orbit. Help from other surgeons such as neurosurgeons, otolaryngology, or maxillofacial surgeons is mandatory in these cases.

3.8. Reconstruction of the exenterated orbit

The decision to reconstruct the exenterated socket depends on what is planned for that orbit. When the patient desires an orbital prosthesis, spontaneous epithelialization, skin grafts, or thin local flaps are good options. Some surgeons argue that spontaneous granulation permits a better follow-up of the cavity in order to treat as soon as possible if disease recurs. Others prefer to fill the cavity with temporalis muscle flap but this increases the difficulty to adapt an orbital prosthesis for the ocularist.

3.9. Spontaneous granulation

It is the fastest way to finish the surgery, and it reduces surgical morbidity in other sites but requires very frequent postsurgical care, initially three times a week and later on every 1 or 2 weeks until complete epithelialization is observed. This can take up to 2 or 3 months more than when split thickness grafts are used. Usually, gauzes with antibiotic ointment are applied in the first month.

3.10. Skin grafting

Split thickness grafts, usually harvested from the thigh with an automated dermatome, are used, which is technically simple to perform and takes less time than a more complex flap reconstruction. In order to adapt the graft to the socket, slits can be performed with scalpel or a number 15 blade. The edges are sutured to the borders of the surgery with absorbable 6/0 sutures. Gauze soaked in antibiotic ointment is packed in the socket, and a pressure dressing is placed for 1 week. Once this is removed, the gauze will be changed every 2 or 3 days until the graft is correctly stuck to the bone beneath.

3.11. Soft tissue reconstruction

Some surgeons advocate primary reconstruction during exenteration surgery. Volume loss in the socket can be replaced with vascularized free flaps. They are useful to cover alloplastic implants or other kind of flaps used for bony reconstruction. One of their disadvantages is donor site morbidity. Another one is that aesthetics in the donor site and the socket may seem unnatural. Many local flaps have been used, including temporoparietal fascia, temporalis muscle, or frontalis muscle. As said previously, these flaps can potentially affect postoperative tumor surveillance, making imaging techniques, especially MRI, essential and increasing the cost for the National Health Service or the insurance company. On the other hand, orbital obliteration with a flap reconstruction may confer less pain, improve personal hygiene, and reduce the risk of sino-orbital fistula formation [17]. Spiegel et al [18] reported that orbital obliteration reduces the risk of intracranial infections and facilitates dosage calculation of radiotherapy by providing a more consistent and predictable tissue density.

3.12. Rehabilitation of the socket

Once exenterated, eviscerated, or enucleated, the socket is perceived by the patient and the family as a very significant facial deformity. Initially, the simplest way to mask the socket is with eye patches. However, once the cavity has healed, the patient can benefit from the experience of an ocularist.

Enucleated or eviscerated cavities will have a temporal prosthesis fitted in 4 or 6 weeks after surgery. Later on, a prosthesis will be made using a modified impression technique, so a custom-made prosthesis will be designed and adapted at the ocularist. It is very common that artificial eyes need to be adapted several times after the initial fitting before the patient feels comfortable with them. The patient will be followed at the ocularist once or twice a year to check if the prosthesis fits correctly in the socket, if it is affecting the lower eyelid (the weight of the prosthesis is a key factor) or if its surface needs polishing. The ophthalmologist will check the prosthesis position, the presence or absence of discharge, whether the fornices look normal, how the superior sulcus is, eyelid malpositions, eyelash malposition, relative enophthalmos, etc., when the patient visits the clinic.

Exenterated orbits are more difficult to deal with. Orbital prostheses are made by experienced anaplastologists or ocularists. The material used is completely different, usually silicone. Some patients may find glasses useful to mask the skin silicone interface. Sometimes, especially in shallow orbits, the prosthesis may tend to fall; therefore, magnetic coupling with osseointegrated screws can be fitted in, typically several months after epithelialization of the orbit is complete. Unfortunately, some patients might find that the lack of movement of these prostheses may make other people feel uncomfortable, and prefer to use just an eye patch.

4. Orbital implants

Evisceration and enucleation result in an empty cavity and aesthetic problems for the patients that we should try to avoid. We must be sure that the patient fully understands the information given about the surgery and expected results in order to obtain the informed consent. Once this is done, the surgeon will decide the type of orbital implant, which can be placed primarily or secondarily in another surgery. The implant can be made of synthetic material, autologous material, or eye-banked tissues. The ocularist has a very important role in the aesthetics of the patient. Artificial eyes have enormously improved the psychological impact and the physical image of the person who undergoes this mutilating surgery. It was back in 1885 when Mules suggested the idea of placing orbital implants in these orbits [4]. Later on, Frost used hollow glass spheres as orbital implants. The surgical procedure was slightly modified with time. It was not until 1972 when Soll [19] suggested placing the implant beneath Tenon's capsule. Helveston covered the implant with donor sclera. The volume loss in some sockets, the presence of contracted sockets, or the implant extrusion made Smith and Petrelli propose the use of dermis-fat grafts in some patients. The ideal implant should fulfill these requirements: it should replace enough orbital volume, it should permit the artificial eye to move as much as possible, it should make the eye prosthesis fit adequately in the socket, it should have a low complication rate, it should be cost-effective and simple to implant in the orbit, biocompatible, and it should not degrade [20].

Herein, we will review the available types of implants. Bio-inert and nonporous materials have given way to porous materials. The latter have multiple micropores that are interconnected, mimicking the human bone trabecular meshwork. Complications after orbital implantation will depend on several factors, including the surgical technique, the material and size of the implant, previous orbital treatments (e.g., radiotherapy), orbital disease, poorly fitted artificial eyes, or infections.

4.1. Implant selection

Both evisceration and enucleation can be performed without orbital implants, but nowadays, it is very rare not to use them because of the very poor esthetic results. The goal of placing an implant in the orbit is to compensate the loss of volume, to improve the prosthesis motility, and to offer a good symmetry with the contralateral eye. Some considerations on these facts are as follows:

4.2. Replacing volume loss

Volume loss appears to be the main determinant of anatomic changes after enucleation [21]. Human radiographic studies have confirmed that placing a spherical implant within Tenon's capsule counteracts the rotation of intraorbital contents after enucleation and associated back-tilt of the prosthesis. An adequate volume replacement permits a thinner prosthesis, relieving weight on the lower eyelid and minimizing associated ectropion formation and lid laxity [22]. Furthermore, an inferior displacement of the superior rectus-levator complex is associated to those changes [23]. Therefore, the implant must be big enough to replace the volume loss but not too big, which may create excessive tension on Tenon's capsule that could favor the implant extrusion.

Proper implant size can be calculated either preoperatively (from the axial length of the eye to be operated on or the fellow eye) or intraoperatively (determining the volume of fluid displaced by the enucleated eye in a graduated cylinder). We recommend the first option. Kaltreider et al. [24] showed that the implant diameter should be the eye's axial length minus 2 mm or minus 1 mm if the length was calculated with A-scan. An implant that is too small will need a bigger prosthesis, potentially resulting in lower eyelid laxity and malposition of the artificial eye. Larger than needed implants will require smaller prosthesis but are associated to higher exposure rates and may difficult the adaptation of the artificial eye [25]. We follow the recommendations from Jordan and Klapper for adult patients. These are 20-22 mm spherical implants in enucleation surgery and 18-20 mm spherical implants in evisceration surgery [16].

4.3. Maintaining levator function

Another important issue to consider is the functionality of the levator muscle of the upper lid. The smaller diameter of implant, as compared to the globe alters the functional length and pivot point of the superior rectus-levator complex [26]. These factors may lead to a decreased levator function and ptosis. This situation can be improved either by surgery or by adding to the superior margin of the prosthesis additional material.

We should remember that with time, the orbital tissues of an anophthalmic orbit tend to contract towards the orbital apex, that is, nasally and inferiorly [27].

We can consider orbital implants in two main groups: integrated and nonintegrated implants.

4.4. Nonintegrated implants

They do not have a surface where rectus muscles can be anchored, nor they allow fibrovascular tissue to grow in them (this is why we call them nonintegrated). They include implants made of glass, rubber, iron, acrylic material, silicone, gold, silver, or polymethylmethacrylate [28]. Their only function is to replace the volume loss and to improve the cosmetic result. If the surgeon wants to increase the motility of the implant and, consequently, of the prosthesis, the rectus muscles should be repositioned and sutured to the anterior pole of the implant in order to move the artificial eye when the implant moves. Unfortunately, the movements achieved with this method are of smaller range than dose achieved when the implant is pegged. Some authors have suggested that when the rectus muscles are placed as described previously, that is, in the anterior pole of the implant, it may migrate when the muscles contract. Mourits et al. [29] consider that acrylic implants have a low extrusion rate and are easier to implant and explant (their surface is smoother, and there is no fibrovascular ingrowth to retain the implant) and are cheaper than porous implants. Nonintegrated implants have been widely used and have achieved good results in the end of the 19th century and all over the 20th century. Nowadays, they are still used in patients over 70 years old.

4.5. Integrated implants

4.5.1. Hydroxyapatite

Coralline hydroxyapatite is used frequently in enucleation surgery. It began to be used in orbitary implants in the 1980s. It is a calcium phosphate salt present in the human bone. It is considered to be nontoxic, nonallergenic, and biocompatible. It allows fibrovascular tissue to grow in the implant, thanks to its 3-D architecture [30]. If the fibrovascular growth is poor, there is a risk of implant extrusion. There are two commercially available implants: Bio-Eye (Integrated Orbital Implants, Inc., San Diego, CA) and M-Sphere (IOP, Inc., Costa Mesa, CA). Bio-eye has been the first choice for many surgeons for years. In a survey performed in 2002 with the oculoplastic surgeon members of the American Society of Ophthalmic Plastic and Reconstructive Surgeons (ASOPRS), they inquired about their preferences in primary enucleations; 27.3% used hydroxyapatite while 42.7% used porous polyethylene [31]. Jamell et al. [32] suggested that the best way to evaluate fibrovascular growth into the implant is contrast-enhanced magnetic resonance with surface coil. They were able to show early fibrovascular growth in the implant being the central ingrowth of the fibrovascular tissue slower. This evaluation of the central vascularization of the implant is of great importance in order to know when to peg the implant. The greater vascularized the implant, the bigger the risk of blood when the implant is drilled, but at the same time, it is believed to reduce to the risk of infection, exposure, and migration [32,33]. Nevertheless, this technique has its drawbacks; it is time consuming and expensive. Therefore, sometimes you cannot detect complications of the vascularized implant on time. Due to this, Qi-hua et al. [34] used contrast-enhanced ultrasonography (CEUS) as an alternative to evaluate the implant's vascularization, claiming it is also effective and it is cheaper than the contrast-enhanced MRI. In order to increase the vascularization of the implant, some authors suggest to drill an additional number of holes in the implant where the scleral windows should be before inserting it in the cavity [35]. It is believed that increasing the fibrovascular ingrowth in the implant will decrease its risk of migration and extrusion. It should be emphasized that this type of implant is usually covered with donor sclera or other materials because its rough surface easily erodes the conjunctiva when the implant moves. This coating of the implant is useful to attach the extraocular muscles too. There is synthetic hydroxyapatite, which is half the price of coralline hydroxyapatite. It is easier to drill and to place the peg. There is also bovine hydroxyapatite from the cancellous bone of calf fibulae, fully deproteinized so as to be antigen-free.

When a peg is fit into the implant, this is done 6 or more months after the surgery because this is the time estimated for the vascularization to establish in the implant. This procedure is used in those patients who desire to increase the prosthesis motility.

Complications related to this type of implant are discharge, pyogenic granulomas, loss of the peg, reduced prosthesis motility, and an audible click, which can be annoying for the patient [36]. Calcified hydroxyapatite implants are capable of absorbing radiation. This is of special importance in children that have undergone enucleation surgery secondary to retinoblastoma, as it hinders local recurrences and decreases the effect of secondary orbital irradiation when needed [36-38]. Most patients are satisfied with the cosmetic outcome of the nonpegged implant and do not desire an additional procedure with increased risks for complications.

4.5.2. Porous Polyethylene (MEDPOR)

It is made of synthetic, high-density polyethylene powder. It is flexible and easily moldable in order to adapt it to different shapes [39]. In contrast with hydroxyapatite, it is cheaper, it does not need to be wrapped because the rectus muscles can be tied to it, and it is easier to place in the orbit. Instead of using sutures, some authors have tried to fix the muscles to MEDPOR implants with 2-ocetyl-cyanoacrylate tissue glue [40]. This proof-concept study concluded that this technique seemed safe and had good functional and anatomical results. Porous polyethylene allows fibrovascular ingrowth, but this does not happen as fast as it does in hydroxyapatite. A major drawback of porous polyethylene was that there was no integrating device for the ocular prosthesis available. Shore [41] described a titanium postcoupling system that was included in the implant 6-12 months after the primary surgery. Generally speaking, these implants offer excellent motility, good tolerance, and very few complications. Timoney et al. [42] reported two cases of foreign body inflammatory giant cell reaction in patients who underwent orbital fracture repairs with porous polyethylene implants.

4.5.3. Proplast

This is an alloplastic, biologically inert porous material. It allows fibrovascular ingrowth and attachment of extraocular muscles.

4.5.4. Aluminum oxide

It is a porous ceramic bio-inert material, structurally strong, and free of contaminants. It is cheaper than hydroxyapatite, and its surface is smoother. It is too biocompatible and generates a very mild inflammatory response. It can also be wrapped in Vicryl (polyglactin 910) mesh.

5. Wrapping material

Implant covering improves the volume of the orbit and motility of the prosthesis and provides an additional barrier for the implant. All of these are important factors for an optimal surgical result. It is usually done in nonintegrated implants like silicone but can be used in hydroxyapatite too in order to protect the Tenon's layer and the conjunctiva from the erosion of the rough implant surface.

5.1. Donor sclera

Once warmed up to room temperature, it is advisable to send cultures of the liquid in order to discard any possible microbiological contamination. Sclera is placed over the implant and sutured with 4-0 or 5-0 nonabsorbable running sutures. Due to its origin, there is a small possibility of infection transmission, including human immunodeficiency virus, hepatitis B or C virus, and Creutzfeldt-Jakob disease. These risks have made many surgeons abandon this wrapping material.

5.2. Autologous tissue

This type of tissue includes temporalis fascia, dermis, human donor pericardium, fascia lata, or posterior auricular muscle complex [43]. Their autologous origin prevents an immune host versus graft reaction. Nevertheless, they require an extra surgical procedure to harvest them and prepare them to cover the implant, which increases surgical time, and there is always the risk of donor site morbidity.

5.3. Synthetic tissue

Polyglactin 910 mesh (Vicryl mesh, Ethicon, Sommerville, NJ, USA) is used to wrap hydroxyapatite and bioceramic orbital implants. It offers a series of advantages: there is no risk of disease transmission, there is no need of a second surgical site, and it is easy to use. It has a porous structure that allows fibrovascular ingrowth [33]. Polytetrafluoroethylene and polyglicolic acid (Dexon mesh style no8, Davis & Geck, Manati, Puerto Rico) have also been used as implant cover materials.

Hydroxyapatite polyglactin mesh-wrapped implants [44] have been used in secondary implants with good results both in prosthesis motility and low exposition rate.

6. Considerations in children

The anophthalmic or microphthalmic socket in children has special features that we will discuss. One of the most important issues is that the orbit of the child should continue growing after the eye is removed. The surgeon must have that in mind in order to achieve good cosmetic and anatomical results. This will condition the implant selection.

The most frequent cause of enucleation in pediatric age is retinoblastoma. There has been a special concern whether to place an implant in these orbits due to the difficulties in the follow-up and the detection of tumor recurrence with an orbital implant in place. However, once it was observed that orbits in children with no orbital implants did not develop appropriately, the decision to implant was taken. Normal face and bony orbit growth depends on the orbital soft tissue contents. When the child is five and a half years old, his face is about 90% of the size of an adult's face [45]. Generally talking, the management of an anophthalmic socket in a child younger than 5 years old requires an implant that can increase in size, such as a dermis-fat graft or orbital tissue expander. A large fixed-sized orbital implant can be placed in children older than 5 years [46]. Orbital growth is completed by the time the child is 12-14 years old [47]. Dermis-fat grafts harvested from the thigh have shown to stimulate orbital growth in children [48], but their motility is poor. Thus, this is an ideal implant for children younger than 5 years old. The dermis-fat graft is also used to cover hydroxyapatite exposures and to reconstruct sockets. A low incidence of complications has been reported with hydroxyapatite implants in a large series of pediatric patients who had undergone enucleation surgery for different reasons after 60 months of follow-up and excellent cosmetic results. We should not forget that when treating an anophthalmic cavity in a child, we need to increase the conjunctival fornices, increase the width of the palpebral fissure promoting at the same time the eyelid growth, and expand the orbital bones. These goals can be achieved with a good surgical implant and the use of progressively larger conformers.

Jordan and Klapper recommend choosing the implant depending on several factors. If a child younger than 5 years undergoes enucleation, they choose a 16-18 mm of diameter wrapped nonporous implant (e.g., silicone). They stress that you should introduce the biggest implant that does not create tension when closing the Tenon's and conjunctival layers. Another option may be dermis-fat grafts, knowing that they can reabsorb and loose some of its volume and taking into account that the artificial eye movements will be very limited. In children aged 5-15 years, they recommend hydroxyapatite or aluminum oxide [16]. On the other hand, Shah et al. used hydroxyapatite implants with low complication rates and good motility and high patient/family cosmetic satisfaction on long-term follow-up in 531 orbits of children with an average age of 3 years.

7. Postoperative complications

7.1. Anophthalmic socket complications

We can divide them depending on the surgery performed in the socket.

Patients underwent enucleation or evisceration.

7.1.1. Dryness, discharge, or irritation

Tear secretion may decrease with time [50]. Patients may be advised to use artificial tears or gel. Saline solution can be used to clean the ocular surface. Most anophthalmic sockets have some degree of discharge. Foreign body reaction, loss of prosthetic surface polishing, and therefore smooth surface, abrasion of conjunctival surface, and accumulation of debris between the prosthesis and the conjunctiva are factors that are believed to increase the production of debris and discharge [51]. It is advisable to minimize the handling of the prosthesis. If discharge is present, both the socket and the prosthesis should be evaluated. Scratches and loss of luster are relatively frequent, especially if the prosthesis is old. The ocularist usually helps with keeping the surface polished by smoothing the surface and removing proteins and debris every 6 or 12 months. Once surface problems or inadequate fit in the socket have been discarded, steroid or antibiotic steroid drops can be used once or twice daily. If the discharge is mucopurulent, especially if the eyelids are swollen and conjunctival hyperemia and chemosis is present, an infectious conjunctivitis should be considered. Treatment should include cultures and antibiotic (quinolone) drops.

Some patients may have a giant papillary conjunctivitis, which may require steroid and antihistamine drops. The artificial eye should be removed in the night and washed in soft contact lens daily cleaner and denture cleaning products.

7.1.2. Pain

Pain after eye removal is difficult to handle. If the prosthesis is correctly fit in the orbit, the conjunctiva should be checked for any signs of inflammation or infection. If the implant migrates anteriorly, it can compress the tissue and hurt. Pain may have its origin in the trochlea. This can be examined by pressing on this zone. If the pain resembles that experienced by the patient, triamcinolone injection in the trochlea can be effective [52]. Other causes or pain may be amputation neuroma, sinus inflammation, tumor, depression, or secondary gain [53].

7.1.3. Orbital cysts

They manifest as pain or pressure sensation or even only increased difficulty to fit the artificial eye. Cysts may grow if conjunctival epithelium is incarcerated after wound closure or when there is epithelial ingrowth in wound dehiscence [54]. Management options are complete surgical excision, marsupialization, absolute alcohol injection, or trichloroacetic acid (TCA) injection [55].

7.1.4. Lower eyelid malposition

When the eye is enucleated, the disruption of the fibrous framework of the orbit may result in the rotation of the orbital contents inferiorly and anteriorly. This will shallow the inferior fornix and tilt the prosthesis. The inferior portion of the prosthesis pushes on the inferior eyelid, while the superior portion moves posteriorly inside the orbit, deepening the superior sulcus. Both of these two features are part of the anophthalmic socket syndrome, which includes an upper eyelid ptosis, a deep superior sulcus, an enophthalmos, a lower eyelid malposition, and a fornix retraction. With time, the lower eyelid becomes more lax, especially when heavier prosthesis is fitted. This enhances the inferior migration of orbital tissues. The final result is a poorly fitting artificial eye, lower eyelid malposition, shortening of the inferior fornix, and deepening of the superior sulcus. In older patients, the laxity of the inferior eyelid increases, especially when wearing a prosthesis even if it is not heavy.

7.2. Eyelash misdirection and entropion

Several situations are responsible for eyelash misdirection. Fornix contracture is one of the most common due to the trauma of surgery of the eye removal or contracture as a result of chemical burn. Sometimes the contracture of the fornix is result of the contracture of the conjunctiva as a result of chronic inflammation. Lower eyelid laxity can also produce eyelash misdirection. In order to correct eyelash misdirection, there are a series of options depending on the underlying cause. When laxity of the eyelid is present, lateral canthoplasty can be a good option. A transverse tarsal incision with marginal rotation is a simple way to change the direction of the eyelashes. If there is a shallow fornix, a silicone band to reform the fornix is a suitable option, but if there is a moderate to severe contraction of the fornix, fornix deepening will require grafts that may be harvested from the hard palate, ear cartilage, or contralateral upper lid tarsus.

7.2.1. Ectropion

It is normally associated to lower eyelid laxity with aging in normal anophthalmic sockets. Heavy prosthesis or frequent removal of the artificial eye will result in premature ectropion, sometimes in very young patients. If the enucleation was due to orbital and eye trauma, skin scars can precipitate the apparition of ectropion. When ectropion is due to eyelid laxity, lateral tarsal strip is a good and a simple surgical option that offers good results. Heavy prosthesis should be changed for lighter ones. Anterior lamella contraction should be treated with skin or skin and muscle grafts and may benefit from lateral canthopexy procedures to tighten the eyelid.

7.2.2. Ptosis

Ptosis in an anophthalmic socket is sometimes difficult to manage. Too small or too big implants, migration of the implant, levator traumatic damage, trauma from a poorly fitted prosthesis, trauma from the original injury, or levator aponeurosis dehiscence from the tarsal plate can end in upper eyelid ptosis. If the implant is too small, it can be replaced for a bigger one or volume can be increased with a dermis-fat graft. When the implant migrates inferior and anteriorly, it can be repositioned superior and posteriorly with a subperiosteal implant. Once the other factors have been considered and corrected if possible, a levator aponeurosis advancement can be achieved through an anterior approach. The anterior approach will preserve the conjunctiva from potentially contract and helps to create a symmetric eyelid crease.

7.2.3. Deep superior sulcus and enophthalmos

Soft tissue and volume changes in the socket after enucleation or evisceration are responsible of upper lid ptosis and lower lid laxity but also deepening of the superior sulcus. Even when the initial surgical result may be satisfactory, with time, the implant may migrate inferior and anteriorly, deepening the superior sulcus and making the eye socket look sunken or enophthalmic. Conservative management may include alterations in the prosthesis or wearing glasses to camouflage the superior sulcus. Best results should be expected with surgery. Volume augmentation with orbital floor implant placement is the first step, followed by superior sulcus fat grafting and lower lid tightening. The last surgical procedure will be ptosis repair.

Orbital floor implants placed subperiosteally are indicated if the implant is of adequate size and in position. Different materials such as acrylic (polymethylmethacrylate), bone grafts, hydroxyapatite, autogenous fat, injectable hydroxyapatite, dermis-fat grafts, and others have been used. Polymethylmethacrylate is a well-tolerated material placed subperiosteally using a swinging eyelid technique. This implant displaces the orbital implant and surrounding connective tissue and fat anterior and superiorly, thus reducing the sunken superior sulcus. If there is a residual defect after this surgery or when the defect of the superior sulcus is mild or when the patients rejects the placement of a subperiosteal implant, the superior sulcus can be filled with a dermis-fat graft or with an autologous fat graft or a dermal filler such as hyaluronic acid [56]

7.2.4. Implant exposure or extrusion

They are the most frequent complications reported in the literature. They can happen with any kind of implant and at any time. There are many factors involved, including incorrect closure of the wound, infections, implant too large for the socket, bad prosthesis adaptation, or delayed fibrovascular ingrowth.

Exposures in the first 3 months after the surgery are probably due to poor wound healing or surgical closure or incorrect position of the orbital implant. Once again, we would like to highlight the importance of a correct tension-free closure of Tenon's layer. Exposures occurring 3 months to 1 year after surgery can be due to the factors previously reported and others like infection or inflammatory response. When exposures occur beyond the first 2 years, they are usually due to mechanical factors such as friction or pressure from the prosthesis [57].

If a nonporous implant exposition is acute and not too big, it can be solved with prompt medical or surgical treatment, but when the exposition is big (more than 3 mm) or long lasting (4 months or more), it usually leads to implant extrusion and, therefore, to its removal. On the other hand, exposed porous implants generally do not extrude because of their fibrovascular anchorage in the socket [58]. Although some porous implants can expose 10 years after surgery, most of the exposures take place within the first year after the surgery. As mentioned above, the use of materials that cover porous implants is an attempt to reduce implant exposition when the surface of the implant is rough enough to rub and tear the conjunctiva. However, Suter et al. [59] have suggested that this kind of material could produce the contrary effect as it would act as a barrier to fibrovascular ingrowth. Kamai et al. [60] used 20% autologous serum when there was conjunctival postoperative dehiscence and necrosis with good results. They recommend to put a drop at least 10 times a day. They observed that the healing occurred after 2 weeks of autologous serum use, preventing the exposure of the implant. Quaranta-Leoni et al. [61] found the presence of Gram-positive cocci infection in 59% of the patients in a group of 25 people when the porous orbital implants were exposed requiring explantation. A histopathological examination showed the presence of a chronic inflammatory infiltrate in 22 implants (88%) and significantly reduced fibrovascular ingrowth of the implant in all patients. They considered a good surgical option the implantation of a dermis-fat graft in the socket once explanted the implant in order to address the volume deficit following implant removal.

There are many surgical options to treat exposed implants: scleral patch grafts [62], mucous membrane grafts [63], temporalis fascia grafts [64], conjunctival pedicle grafts [65], and dermis-fat grafts [66]. Chu et al. [67] proposed a triple layer to treat exposed implants: donor sclera, muscle flaps, and oral mucosa.

7.2.5. Socket contracture

The patient will complain that the prosthesis keeps falling out of the socket. Acquired socket contraction is the consequence of shrinkage and shortening of some or all of the tissues of the anophthalmic orbit; thus, the fornices are not able to retain the prosthesis. In order to prevent it, it is mandatory to carry out a straightforward enucleation or evisceration surgery that is, taking care to keep trauma to the conjunctiva, connective tissue, and orbital at minimum levels.

Fornices should not be undermined, and cauterization should be minimized by using gauzes soaked in freezing water and using the bipolar cautery with low energy levels. The conformer should be fit in the socket once the surgery is finished and kept in place until a nondefinite artificial eye is fitted [68]. The more surgeries a socket undergoes, the bigger the risk of developing a socket contracture. In order to simplify its management, we can classify it into the following:

Mild socket contracture. When the posterior lamella shortens, the lashes rotate inward and entropion develops. There is a decrease of the inferior fornix causing a prolapse of the inferior pole of the prosthesis. A transverse tarsal incision with marginal rotation is the initial treatment of choice [69]. There is usually a lower eyelid horizontal laxity too. When there is enough conjunctiva, a lateral canthal tendon procedure associated to a fornix reformation procedure should be performed. The fornix is reformed using 3-0 or 4-0 polyglactin sutures anchored to the periorbita and skin tied over a bolster [70]. However, if there is a lower lid contraction, a posterior lamella lengthening procedure is the best option. Several autogenous spacer grafts have been used: fascia lata, oral mucosa [71], nasal cartilage, hard palate, upper eyelid tarsus, or auricular cartilage [72]. Auricular cartilage is easy to harvest, provides support for the artificial eye, lengthens the posterior lamella, and prevents forward tilt of the prosthesis [73]. Oral mucosa is an excellent option to increase the mucous surface but lacks supportive properties.

Moderate socket contracture. One or both of the fornices are contracted. Typically, the first to contract is the inferior fornix. When the superior fornix contracts, the artificial eye may be retained but the eyelid excursion may be very limited. The gold standard for the treatment of moderate socket contracture is mucous membrane grafting, usually obtained from oral (lip) or buccal (cheek) mucosa [74,75]. Grafts undergo shrinkage with time, so a graft harvested 40% bigger than the defect is recommended. The conjunctiva is undermined, and the graft is sutured with absorbable 7-0 interrupted sutures. A retinal band can be used to reform the inferior and upper fornices, anchoring it to the periorbita and the skin with bolsters. Then a conformer is placed. Amniotic membrane has also been used as a graft with good results.

If the patient has a socket volume deficiency associated to the socket contracture, the patient will improve with a dermis-fat graft [76], increasing the orbital volume and the conjunctival surface area.

Severe socket contracture. The conjunctival fornices are nearly or completely obliterated, and the prosthesis may fall constantly or give the patient a "staring" appearance. It is frequent to have discharge and irritation or even an active inflammation. The goal of the surgery is to make the patient comfortable and have a good cosmesis. The patient may need to undergo several surgeries with buccal mucosa grafts and flaps from temporalis muscle or radial forearm. When results are very poor, some patients may benefit from an exenteration procedure, which may improve the aesthetics and the comfort of the socket.

Patients underwent exenteration.

7.3. Exenterated orbit

7.3.1. Sino-orbital fistula

Its frequency has been reported to be as high as 68% [77] and as low as 28% [78]. It is more common when the orbit is left to granulate rather than when a skin graft is used. The majority affect the ethmoid sinus. Risk factors are surgical trauma to the ethmoid or lacrimal bones, sinus disease, radiotherapy, and immunocompromised. They can lead to ethmoidal sinusitis. Management ranges from conservative socket hygiene to surgical repair with flaps or grafts, but it is not unusual for the fistula to recur [79].

7.3.2. Chronic discharge

Once healed, if the socket has a sino-orbital fistula, pus from the ethmoid sinus can drain to the orbit when sinusitis is present. In these cases, systemic antibiotics like third-generation cephalosporin twice daily for 14 days may be enough. If medical treatment is not curative, the patient may be referred to the head and neck surgeon in order to program the patient for endoscopic sinus drainage surgery.

The skin coating the orbit will need to be cleaned with soap and water, just as any other part of the body. Sometimes patients are reticent to let anyone do this for them and it is relatively frequent to find dirty skin in the orbit.

7.3.3. Cerebrospinal fluid leak

A cerebrospinal fluid (CSF) leak may lead to meningitis, delayed cerebral abscess, seizures, CSF hypotension with position-dependent headache syndrome, occult hemorrhage, and even death [80]. The incidence reported by an Australian team was 0.6% [81]. However, it can be as high as 29% [82]. Interestingly, the intraoperative use of monopolar cautery in areas of thin orbital bone may contribute to the incidence of CSF leaks [83]. Once you detect clear liquid leaking from the bone in areas of high risk of encountering dura, prompt treatment usually ends in good results. It is very advisable to consult the neurosurgery team. A dural laceration can be sutured with 5-0 or 6-0 polyglactin or nylon to create a watertight seal. If the defect is large, an autologous graft (fat, temporalis muscle or fascia, and pericranium) and a tissue adhesive such as human fibrinogen and bovine thrombin or cyanoacrylate [84] can be used. In smaller defects, tissue adhesives may be enough to seal the leak. Additional materials used in the repair of CSF leaks at other sites include the use of gelfoam® in epidural blood patches. At the end, packing material can be placed in the socket to hold the plug of muscle or fascia against the defect and therefore protect from further leakage. After surgery, the patient must avoid blowing his or her nose and coughing as well as physical activity. Acetazolamide is used to reduce the production of CSF in order to treat CSF leaks. Some authors use systemic antibiotics when there is an intraoperative leak of CSF, but many believe they are unnecessary to prevent meningitis [85].

7.3.4. Delayed healing

The orbital defect left to heal spontaneously once exenterated will granulate slowly if allowed only to grow from the orbital rim, and it will heal faster when it heals from spared eyelids. Nevertheless, this will take at least 2-3 months more than when the defect is covered by a temporalis muscle transposition [86], dermis-fat graft (in subtotal exenteration), or split skin graft [87]. Healing by granulation has shorter operating room time and allows for better clinical monitoring of recurrence. However, it requires frequent visits to change the dressings [88], every week and sometimes every 2 or 3 days, and may delay other therapeutic procedures such as radiotherapy. Depending on how the granulation process is developing, dressings may need to be associated to hydrogel mesh or silver mesh. Orbital obliteration with temporalis muscle or a graft may induce less pain, improve personal hygiene, and reduce the risk of sino-orbital fistula, but it requires image techniques such as MRI, CT, or PET to detect local recurrences.

7.3.5. Tumor recurrence

Tumor recurrence following orbital exenteration can occur in 24-45% of cases [82,89]. Early detection of tumor recurrence in patients who have undergone orbital exenteration is very important. This task is relatively easy when the orbit was left to granulate, but it is difficult when the normal anatomical landmarks have been lost (like when exenteration is associated to ethmoidectomy), and there are flaps covering large cavities. Recurrent tumors may appear as soft tissue similar to the primary tumor, especially in the first 2 years of the surgery (65% of the cases) and in the margin of the flap [90]. Lee et al. recommend to follow this patients with frequent MRI, at least every 4 months after surgery for the 2 first years and every 6 months for 3 more years. On MRI, recurrences appear on the margin of the flap and are often T2 isointense, as opposed to the hyperintense appearance described in normal flaps. PET has also been used to help to differentiate recurrence from scarring or radiation-associated tissue changes.

8. Conclusions

The removal of the eye in any surgical variants (enucleation, evisceration, and exenteration) requires a careful and thorough planning process. A detailed patient explanation of the causes that have led to this type of surgery is mandatory as a breakdown of the consequences of the operation. These explanations should be extended to the family as the immediate aesthetic impact not only affects the patient. Once the most appropriate surgical technique has been chosen, it should be planned in detail beforehand, including potential needs for collaboration with other surgical specialties such as plastic surgery, maxillofacial surgery, neurosurgery, or otolaryngology. It is also important to have the support of anesthesiology for good intraoperative monitoring of the patient. The surgical procedure must be done with thoroughness and patience since the surgical time is long in many cases, and rigorous performance of the surgical steps is one factor that decreases the rate of complications. In cases where an implant is required, this can be carried out in a primary or secondary way. The advantages and disadvantages of different types of implants and the use of wrapping material is widely discussed with the patient. It is important to emphasize the patient-recovering milestones and possible postoperative complications as well as the need for other secondary surgical techniques, e.g., eyelid surgery. Postoperative follow-up is crucial to detect and treat complications as early as possible. Finally, we would like to stress that collaboration with the ocularist is essential in order to get a good adaptation of the prosthesis and aesthetical patient satisfaction.

Author details

César Hita-Antón[1], Lourdes Jordano-Luna[2,3] and Rosario Díez-Villalba[2,3*]

*Address all correspondence to: mdiez.hugf@salud.madrid.org

1 Department of Ophthalmology, Hospital Universitario de Torrejón, Torrejón de Ardoz, Madrid, Spain

2 Department of Ophthalmology Hospital Universitario de Getafe, Getafe, Madrid, Spain

3 Universidad Europea de Madrid, Madrid, Spain

References

[1] Kübler-Ross E. On Death and Dying. Macmillan New York; 1969.

[2] Meltzer MA, Schaefer DP, Della Rocca RC. Evisceration. Smith's Ophthalmic Plastic and Reconstructive Surgery. Vol. 2. St. Louis: CV Mosby; 1987. pp. 1300-1307.

[3] Noyes W. Treatise on Diseases of the Eye. New York: Wodd; 1881. p. 189.

[4] Mulles PH. Evisceration of the globe, with artificial vitreous. Transactions of the Ophthalmological Societies of the United Kingdom 1885;5:200-206.

[5] Frost WA. What is the best method of dealing with a lost eye? British Medical Journal 1887:1153.

[6] Hansen AB, Petersen C, Heegaard S. Review of 1028 bulbar eviscerations and enucleations: changes in etiology and frequency overall 20 year period. Acta Ophthalmologica Scandinava. 1999;77:331-335.

[7] Levine MR, Pou CR, Lash RH. Evisceration: is sympathetic ophthalmia a concern in the new millennium? Ophthalmic Plastic and Reconstructive Surgery 1999;15:4.

[8] Alino AM, Perry HD, Kanellopoulos AS, Donnenfeld ED, Rahn EK. Conjunctival flaps. Ophthalmology 1998;105:1120-3.

[9] Massry GG, Holds JB. Evisceration with scleral modification. Ophthalmic Plastic and Reconstructive Surgery 2001;17:42-47.

[10] Ozgur OR, Levent A, Dogan OK. Primary implant placement with evisceration in patients with endophthalmitis. American Journal of Ophthalmology 2007;143:902-904.

[11] Nassab Rs, Thomas SS, Murray D. Orbital exenteration for advanced periorbital skin cancers. 20 years of experience. Journal of Plastic, Reconstructive and Aesthetic Surgery 2007;60:1103-1109.

[12] Levin PS, Dutton JJ. A 20 years series orbital exenteration. American Journal of Ophthalmology 1991;112:496-501.

[13] Collins GL, Nickoonahand N, Morgan MB. Changing demographics and pathology of non-melanoma skin cancer in the last 30 years. Seminars in Cutaneous Medicine and Surgery 2004;23(1):80-83.

[14] Nerad JA, Enucleation, evisceration, and exenteration. The care of the eye socket. In: Nerad JA (Ed.), Techniques in Ophthalmic Plastic Surgery. Elsevier. pp. 463-486.

[15] Sales-Sanz M, Sanz-Lopez A. Four-petal evisceration: a new technique. Ophthalmic Plastic and Reconstructive Surgery 2007;23(5):389-392.

[16] Jordan DR, Klapper SR. Enucleation, evisceration, secondary orbital implantation. In: Black E, Nesi F, Calvano C, Gladstone G, Levine M (Eds). Smith and Nesi's Ophthalmic Plastic and Reconstructive Surgery. New York: Springer; 2011. pp. 1105-1130.

[17] Yeatts R. The esthetics of orbital exenteration. American Journal of Ophthalmology 2005;139:152-153.

[18] Spiegel J, Varvares M. Prevention of postexenteration complications by obliteration of the orbital cavity. Skull Base 2007;17:197-203.

[19] Soll DB. Donor sclera in enucleation surgery. Archives of Ophthalmology 1974;92:494-495.

[20] Chalasani R, Poole-Warren L, Conway RM, Ben-Nissan B. Porous orbital implants in enucleation: a systematic review. Survey of Ophthalmology 2007;52:145-155.

[21] Smit TJ, Koorneef L, Zonneveld FW, Groet E, Otto AJ. Primary and secondary implants in the anophthalmic orbit. Preoperative and postoperative computed tomographic appearance. Ophthalmology 1991;98:106-110.

[22] Sami D, Young S, Petersen S. Perspective on orbital enucleation implants. Survey of Ophthalmology 52:244-265, 2007.

[23] Smit TJ, Koornneef L, Zonneveld FW, Groet E, Otto AJ. Computed tomography in the assessment of the postenucleation socket syndrome. Ophthalmology 97:1347-1351, 1990.

[24] Kaltreider SA, Jacobs JL, Hughes MO. A simple algorithm for selection of implant size for enucleation and evisceration. Ophthalmic Plastic and Reconstructive Surgery 2002;18:336-42.

[25] Thaller VT. Enucleation volume measurement. Ophthalmic Plastic and Reconstructive Surgery 1997;13:18-20.

[26] Tyers AG, Collin JR. Orbital implants and post enucleation socket syndrome. Transactions of the Ophthalmological Societies of the United Kingdom 1982;102:90-92.

[27] Moshfeghi DM, Moshfeghi AA, Finger PT. Enucleation. Survey of Ophthalmology 2000;44:277-301.

[28] Beard C. Remarks on historical and newer approaches to orbital implants. Ophthalmic Plastic and Reconstructive Surgery 1995;11:89-90.

[29] Mourits DL, Hartong DT, Moll AC, Mourits MP. Management of porous orbital implants requiring explantation: a clinical and histopathology study. Letters to the Editor. Ophthalmic Plastic and Reconstructive Surgery 2014;30:528.

[30] Ferrone PJ, Dutton JJ. Rate of vascularization of coralline hydroxyapatite ocular implants. Ophthalmology 1992;99:376-379.

[31] Su GW, Yen MT. Current trends in managing the anophthalmic socket after primary enucleation and evisceration. Ophthalmic Plastic and Reconstructive Surgery 2004;20:274-280.

[32] Jamell GA, Hollsten DA, Hawes MJ, et al. Magnetic resonance imaging versus bone scan for assessment of vascularization of the hydroxyapatite orbital implant. Ophthalmic Plastic and Reconstructive Surgery 1996;12:127-130.

[33] Klapper SR, Jordan D, Punja K, et al. Hydroxyapatite implant wrapping materials: analysis of fibrovascular ingrowth in an animal model. Ophthalmic Plastic and Reconstructive Surgery 2000;16:278-85.

[34] Qi-hua X, Chen Z, Jian-gang Z, Da-zhong Z, Yong-qiang Z. Comparison of contrast-enhanced ultrasonography and contrast-enhanced MRI for the assessment of vascularization of hydroxyapatite orbital implants. Clinical Imaging 2014;38:616-620.

[35] Dutton JJ. Advances and controversies in ophthalmic plastic surgery: enucleation and evisceration. The 1998 American Academy of Ophthalmology Annual Meeting, New Orleans, LA, November 10, 1998.

[36] Jordan DR, Chan S, Mawn L, Gilbert S, Dean T, Brownstein S, Hill VE. Complications associated with pegging hydroxyapatite orbital implants. Ophthalmology 1999;106:505-512.

[37] Karcioglu ZA, Al-Ghamdi H, Al-Bateri A, Rostem A. Radiation absorption properties of orbital implants. Orbit 1998;17:161-167.

[38] Arora V, Weeks K, Halperin EC, Dutton JJ. Influence of coralline hydroxyapatite used as an ocular implant on the dose distribution of external beam photon radiation therapy. Ophthalmology 1992;99:380-382.

[39] Karesh JW, Dresner SC. High-density porous polyethylene (MEDPOR) as a successful anophthalmic socket implant. Ophthalmology 1994;101:1688-1695, discussion 1695-1696.

[40] Warder D, Kratky V. Fixation of extraocular muscles to porous orbital implants using 2-ocetyl-cyanoacrylate glue. Ophthalmic Plastic and Reconstructive Surgery 2014; Oct 10. [Epub ahead of print].

[41] Shore JW. Porous polyethylene orbital implants. The 18 American Academy of Ophthalmology Annual, New Orleans, LA, November 10, 1998.

[42] Timoney PJ, Clark JD, Frederick PA, Krakauner M, Compton C, Horbinski C, Sokol J, Nunery WR. Foreign body granuloma following orbital reconstruction with porous polyethylene. Ophthalmic Plastic and Reconstructive Surgery 2014; Nov 12. [Epub ahead of print].

[43] Naugle TC, Lee AM, Halk BG, Callahan MA. Wrapping hydroxyapatite orbital implants with posterior auricular muscle complex grafts. American Journal of Ophthalmology 199;128:495-501.

[44] Quarante-Leoni FM, Sposanto S, Lorenzano D. Secondary orbital ball implants after enucleation evisceration: surgical management, morbidity, and long-term outcome. Ophthalmic Plastic and Reconstructive Surgery 2014 Jul 14. [Epub ahead of print].

[45] Farkas LG, Posnick JC, Hreczko TM, Pron GE. Growth patterns in the orbital region: a morphometric study. Cleft Palate-Craniofacial Journal 1992;29:315-318.

[46] Chen D, Heher K. Management of the anophthalmic socket in pediatric patients. Current Opinion in Ophthalmology 2004;15:449-453.

[47] Furuta M. Measurement of orbital volume by computed tomography: especially on the growth of the orbit. Japanese Journal of Ophthalmology 200;104:724-728.

[48] Katowitz JA. Orbital expansion with dermis-fat graft in the pediatric age group. Presented at the annual meeting of the American Academy of Ophthalmology, Anaheim, California, October 14, 1991.

[49] Shah SU, Shields CL, Lally SE, Shields JA. Hydroxyapatite orbital implant in children following enucleation: analysis of 531 sockets. Ophthalmic Plastic and Reconstructive Surgery 2014; Jun 3. [Epub ahead of print].

[50] Larned DC. Lacrimal mechanics in the enucleated state. Ophthalmic Plastic and Reconstructive Surgery 1992;8:202-207.

[51] Vasquez RJ, Lindberg JV. The anophthalmic socket and prosthetic eye: a clinical and bacteriological study. Ophthalmic Plastic and Reconstructive Surgery 1989;5:277-280.

[52] Jordan DR. Experience with 130 synthetic hydroxyapatite implants (FCI3). Ophthalmic Plastic and Reconstructive Surgery 2001;17 (3):184-190.

[53] Jordan DR, Brownstein S, Dorey MW. Clinicopathologic analysis of 15 explanted hydroxyapatite implants. Ophthalmic Plastic and Reconstructive Surgery 2004;20(4): 285-290.

[54] McCarthy RW, Beyer CK, Dallow, et al. Conjunctival cysts of the orbit following enucleation. Ophthalmology 1981;88:30-35.

[55] Sanchez EM, Formento NA, Peres-Lopez M, Jimenez AA. Role of trichloroacetic acid in treating posterior conjunctival cystin anophthalmic socket. Orbit 2009;28:101-103.

[56] Morley AMS, Taban M, Malhorta R, Goldberg R. Use of hyaluronic acid gel for upper eyelid filling and contouring. Ophthalmic Plastic and Reconstructive Surgery 2009;25:440-444.

[57] Jordan DR, Klapper SR, Gilberg SM, Dutton JJ, Wong A, Mawn L. The bioceramic implant: evaluation of implant exposures in 419 implants. Ophthalmic Plastic and Reconstructive Surgery 2010:26;80-82.

[58] Custer PL, Kennedy RH, Woog JJ, Kaltreider SA, Meyer DR. Orbital implants in enucleation surgery. A report by the American Academy of Ophthalmology. Ophthalmology 2003;110:2054-2061.

[59] Suter AJ, Molteno AC, Bevin TH, Fulton JD, Herbison P. Long term follow up of bone derived hydroxyapatite orbital implants. British Journal of Ophthalmology 2002;86:1287-1292.

[60] Kamai S, Kumar S, Goer R. Autologous serum for anterior tissue necrosis after porous orbital implant. Middle East African Journal of Ophthalmology 2014;21:193-195.

[61] Quarante-Leoni FM, Moretti C, Sposanto S, Nardoni S, Lambiase A, Bonini S. Management of porous orbital implants requiring explantation: a clinical and histopathological study. Ophthalmic Plastic and Reconstructive Surgery 2014;30:132-136.

[62] Inkster CF, Ng SG, Leatherbarrow B Primary banked scleral patch graft in the prevention of exposure of hydroxyapatite orbital implants. Ophthalmology 2002;109:389-392.

[63] Lee-Wing MW. Amniotic membrane for repair of exposed hydroxyapatite orbital implant. Ophthalmic Plastic and Reconstructive Surgery 2003;19:401-402.

[64] Sagoo MS, Olver JM. Autogenous temporalis fascia patch graft for porous polyethylene (MEDPOR) sphere orbital implant exposure. British Journal of Ophthalmology 2004;88:942-946.

[65] Lu L, Shi W, Luo M, Sun Y, Fan X. Repair of exposed hydroxyapatite orbital implants by subconjunctival tissue flaps. Journal of Craniofacial Surgery 2011;22:1452-1456.

[66] Lee BJ, Lewis CD, Perry JD. Exposed porous orbital implants treated with simultaneous secondary implant and dermis fat graft. Ophthalmic Plastic and Reconstructive Surgery 2010;26:273-276.

[67] Chu HY, Liao YL, Tsai YJ, Chu YC, Wu SY, Ma L. Use of extraocular muscle flaps in the correction of orbital implant exposure. PLoS One. 2013 Sep 25;8(9):e72223. doi: 10.1371/journal.pone.0072223. eCollection 2013.

[68] Tawfik HA, Raslan AO, Talib N. Surgical management of acquired socket contracture. Current Opinion in Ophthalmology 2009;20:406-11.

[69] Kersten RC. Kleiner FP, Kulwin DR. Tarsotomy for the treatment of cicatricial entropion with trichiasis. Archives of Ophthalmology 1992;110:714-7.

[70] Ma'luf RN. Correction of the inadequate lower fornix in the anophthalmic socket. British Journal of Ophthalmology 1999;83:881-2.

[71] Molgat YM, Hurwitz JJ, Webb MC. Buccal mucous membrane fat graft in the management of the contracted socket. Ophthalmic Plastic and Reconstructive Surgery 1993;9:267-72.

[72] Jackson IT, Dubin B, Harris J. Use of contoured and stabilized conchal cartilage grafts for lower eyelid support: a preliminary report. Plastic and Reconstructive Surgery 1989;83:636-40.

[73] Smith RJ, Malet T. Auricular cartilage grafting to correct lower conjunctival fornix retraction and eyelid malposition in anophthalmic patients. Ophthalmic Plastic and Reconstructive Surgery 2008;24(1):13-8.

[74] Klein M, Mennekin H, Bier J. Reconstruction of the contracted ocular socket with free full thickness mucous membrane graft. International Journal of Oral and Maxillofacial Surgery 2000;29:96-8.

[75] Bowen EJ, Nunes E. The outcome of oral mucosal grafts to the orbit: a three and a half year study. British Journal of Plastic Surgery 2002;55:100-4.

[76] Betharia SM, Patil ND. Dermis fat grafting in contracted sockets. Indian Journal of Ophthalmology 1988;36:110-2.

[77] Mohr C, Esser J. Orbital exenteration: surgical and reconstructive strategies. Graefe's Archive for Clinical and Experimental Ophthalmology 1997;235:288-95.

[78] Rahman I, Cook AE, Leatherbarrow B. Orbital exenteration: a 13 year Manchester experience. British Journal of Ophthalmology 2005;89:1335-40.

[79] Limawararut V, Leibovitch I, Davis G, Rees G, Goldberg R, Selva D. Sino-orbital fistula: a complication of exenteration. Ophthalmology 2007;114(2):355-361.

[80] Ebersold M. Five things oculoplastic surgeons should know about neurosurgery. Ophthalmic Plastic and Reconstructive Surgery 2000;16:247-9.

[81] Limawararut V, Valenzuela AA, Sullivan TJ, McNab AA, Malhotra R, Davis G, Jones N, Selva D. Cerebrospinal fluid leaks in orbital and lacrimal surgery. Survey in Ophthalmology. 2008;53(3):274-284.

[82] Kuo CH, Gao K, Clifford A, Shannon K, Clark J. Orbital exenterations: an 18-year experience from a single head and neck unit. ANZ Journal of Surgery 2011 May;81(5): 326-30.

[83] Wulc AE, Adams JL, Dryden RM. Cerebrospinal fluid leakage complicating orbital exenteration. Archives of Ophthalmology 1989;107:827-30.

[84] Tse DT, Panje WR, Anderson RL. Cyanoacrylate adhesive used to stop CSF leaks during orbital surgery. Archives of Ophthalmology 1984;102:1337-9.

[85] Yilmazlar S, Arslan E, Kocaeli H, et al. Cerebrospinal fluid leakage complicating skull base fractures: analysis of 81 cases. Neurosurgical Review 2006;29:64-71.

[86] Reese AB, Jones IS. Exenteration of the orbit and repair by transplantation of the temporalis fascia. American Journal of Ophthalmology 1961;51:217-27.

[87] Harting F, Koorneef L, Peeters HJ, Gillissen JP. Glued fixation of split-skin graft to the bony orbit following exenteration. Plastic and Reconstructive Surgery 1985;76:633-5.

[88] Putterman A. Orbital exenteration with spontaneous granulation. Archives of Ophthalmology 1986;104:139-40.

[89] Nemet AY, Martin P, Benger R, et al. Orbital exenteration: a 15-year study of 38 cases. Ophthalmic Plastic and Reconstructive Surgery 2007;23:468-72.

[90] Lee PS, Sedrak P, Guha-Thakurta N, Chang EI, Ginsberg LE, Esmaeli B, Debnam JM. Imaging findings of recurrent tumors after orbital exenteration and free flap reconstruction. Ophthalmic Plastic and Reconstructive Surgery 2014 Jul-Aug;30(4):315-21.

5

New Technologies in Eye Surgery — A Challenge for Clinical, Therapeutic, and Eye Surgeons

Patricia Durán Ospina, Mayra Catalina Cáceres Díaz and Sabrina Lara

Abstract

Eye surgery is always progresses as the same way that the science advances. New emerging technologies such as bio-printing in 3D, developments and mathematical modeling in prototyping lab- on- a chip, visual implants, new biopolymers started to use in eye enucleation, detection of eye biomarkers at the cellular level, bio-sensors and new diagnostic tests should be considered to improve the quality of life of patients after surgery. This chapter provides a review of new and emerging technologies which are already working on global research centers. Emerging and converging technologies are terms used interchangeably to indicate the emergence and convergence of new technologies with demonstrated potential as disruptive technologies. Among them are: nanotechnology, biotechnology, information technology and communication, cognitive science, robotics, and artificial intelligence that have been launched as innovative products that promise to improve the quality of life and vision of patients with ocular compromised or low vision impairment. Some acronyms for these are: NBIC: Nanotechnology, Biotechnology, Information technology and Cognitive science. GNR: Genetics, Nanotechnology and Robotics. GRIN: Genetic, Robotic, Information, and Nanotechnology. BANG: Bits, Atoms, Neurons and Genes. Otherwise, to training ophthalmologist on news techniques, sophisticated simulation machines has been developing around the world.

Keywords: Artificial retina, nanotechnology, visual health, ocular prosthesis, retina

1. Introduction

Eye surgery always progresses the same way as science advances. New emerging technologies such as bio-printing in 3D, mathematical modeling, and developments in prototyping lab-on-a-chip, visual implants, and new biopolymers have started to be used in eye enucleation, the detection of eye biomarkers at the cellular level, bio-sensors, and new diagnostic tests that are considered to improve the quality of life of patients after surgery.

This chapter provides a review of new and emerging technologies, which are already working in global research centers. The term "emerging technologies" refers to the implementation of new innovative products designed to improve the quality of life. Some acronyms used are:

NBIC: Nanotechnology, Biotechnology, Information technology, and Cognitive science.

GNR: Genetics, Nanotechnology, and Robotics.

GRIN: Genetic, Robotic, Information, and Nanotechnology.

BANG: Bits, Atoms, Neurons, and Genes.

New technologies, such as nanotechnology, artificial intelligence, and genetics among others, have emerged not only to create alternatives to health service, but also to provide alternatives for new ophthalmologists in their surgical practice. There are increasing reviews in literature about the relationship with developments such as new surgical techniques not only for refractive surgery but also for simulation prior to cataract. Retina implants incorporating electronic devices, stem cells, and new inserts for corneal implants are some of the many devices made from biopolymers and electronics that have the promise to be an alternative for visually impaired patients.

Otherwise, as a response to training ophthalmologists on these new techniques, sophisticated simulation devices have been developed around the world [1].

2. Problem statement

Eye surgery has always been characterized by innovation, the introduction of new surgical techniques, and also the inclusion of technology. But being so specialized, this information is not readily disclosed to the targeted patients who directly require these new developments in order to restore their vision or improve the quality of their life. Otherwise, medical students and residents in ophthalmology require an overview of these new developments to plan the training for these new techniques and apply it to patients that have these requirements according to the new protocols, inclusion criteria, and the available technology in the operating room in order to plan new investments for clinical practice and training. Knowing where you are in making this progress, communication and the creation of partnerships between experts are priorities to be able to respond to the patients' needs.

This chapter intends to update eye surgeons in new biopolymers and innovations for ocular prostheses and visual implants for visual care. In the previous years, there are a lot of innovations such us visual implants, artificial silicon retinas, suprachoroidal transretinal stimulation (STS), and artificial corneas among others, which are changing nowadays due to the new advancements in technology and also due to the development of new biomaterials, new microelectrodes, and several types of neural devices around the world. Now, real "artificial eyes" are not only the craniofacial, maxillofacial, ocular, and orbital prostheses that replaces an absent eye after an enucleation but they are also new materials such as cryolite glass, gel from cellulose, glass, silicone and porous polyethylene, graphene, dental biopolymers among others that are being implemented as materials for the heart, eye, and other organ implants due to their characteristics to improve good biological compatibility, be more resistant, reduce allergies, and improve durability. These implants are used for the replacement of the orbital content of anophthalmic cavities [2].

The traditional concept of ocular prostheses (ocular, orbital, epithesis, and maxillofacial), visual implants (retinal, optic nerve, cortical, subretinal, epiretinal and cortical), and others of engineering and biomedical sciences have been changing and must be reviewed in the future.

Otherwise, digital cameras, electrodes, and other electronic devices are useful for the visually impaired. In France, there has been some work on retinal implants using nanodiamonds in the artificial retina. This allows converting light signals into electrical signals. In the field of ocular pharmacology, the nanocarrier molecules for the sustained release of drugs and other devices to vitrectomies are some of the significant visual health advancements in the recent years. Additionally, in the field of contact lenses and artificial corneas, biopolymers have been developed for the early detection of keratoconus or systemic diseases. Nanotechnology is emerging as a science applied to the visual industry and medicine, involving a multidiscipli-nary team that requires new directions in the role and performance of ocular professionals around the world in the near future. The handling of materials and processes at the nanoscale (one billionth of a meter) level, the instrumentality in the accurate detection, and the telere-habilitation intervention using robots of bioelectrical retinal implants nano lenses are just some of the promising developments in the field of eye care. Visual health professionals seek the entry of this science in our curricula, research, and training discipline for innovation and technology based on nanotechnology and robotics. The high costs should not prevent the alliance between university research centers and the private industry in bringing innovation to our population and creating transdisciplinary research lines to improve the quality of life in eye health.

In the recent years, we have reviewed scientific literature regarding publications in surgical techniques of eye surgery. The number of publications on visual implants, artificial corneas, stromal rings, and cross linking has increased in the same manner as the development of new patents did. Also in the recent years, the inclusion of digital imaging systems, visual simulators, and virtual and augmented reality, prior or during the surgeries, have taken place. Some of the ophthalmic surgical procedures mentioned above are useful for improving the life quality of patients. This may pose a challenge to ophthalmic surgeons, but, has improved the quality of life of patients and their rehabilitation. The topics are discussed under the following areas: pre-operative tests, operative surgery, prevention of complications and current and future major advances in eye surgery of importance to surgeons, researchers, physicians, and health personnel.

3. Eye surgery on literature

Global announcements regarding new developments in eye surgery across all fields require a systemic search for there are many institutions and authors contributing to this knowledge.

To perform this review, keywords were used: Eye surgery and refractive surgery, eye surgery and visual implants, eye surgery and retinal implants, glaucoma eye surgery, and cataract eye surgery. The resources used were Medline and Scopus criteria for the inclusion of surgical techniques (1990-2014). In this review, it has been noted that many institutions have increased ophthalmology publications in these areas and in recent years, advancements in electronic chips to the retina and visual and retinal implants are growing considerably.

Many eye care research institutes supported by the government and universities from all continents have been working for decades on innovations for eye surgery across all fields (cataract, refractive surgery, stromal rings, and retinal implants), which has been progressing in different countries as evidenced by scientific literature.

Scientific publications related to refractive surgery around the world and the institutes that have most published reports on refractive surgery can be seen in the chart below. Scopus analysis can be useful creating partnerships between researchers in the same field. See Figure 1 [3].

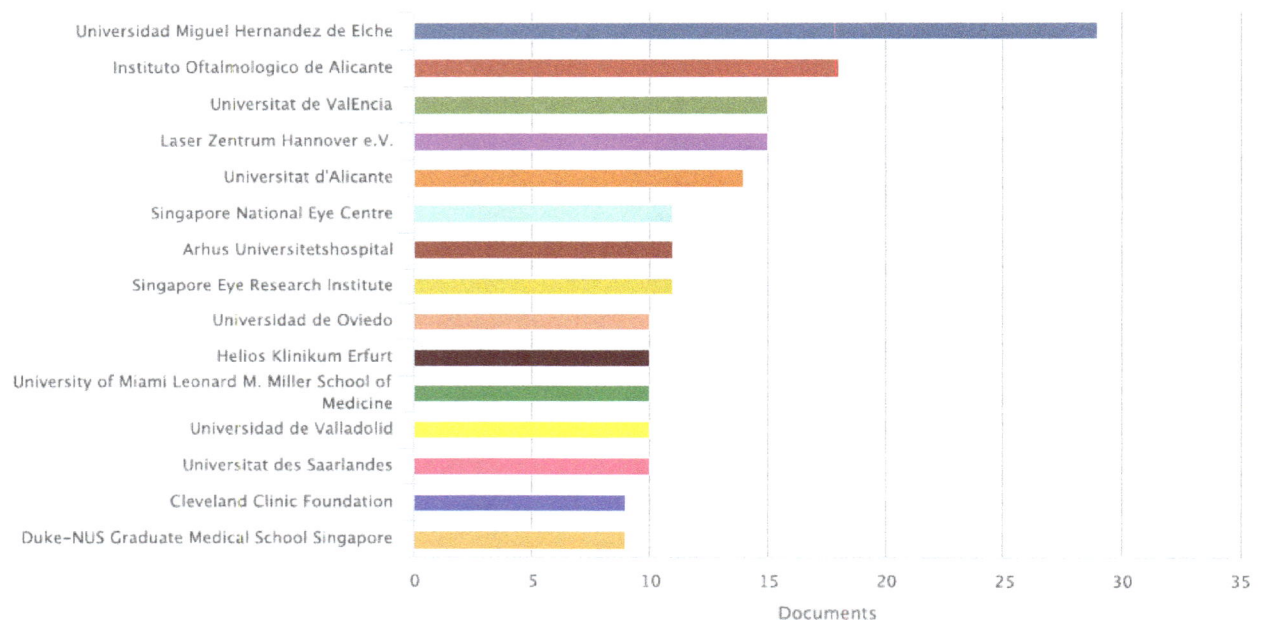

Figure 1. Publications of refractive surgery from Ophthalmology Institutes and Universities around the World from the last decades. Copyright 2015. Elsevier B.V. All right reserved. Scopus is a registered trademark of Elsevier B.V.

Literature reviews on retinal implants, which previously seemed like science fiction, has become a research field not only in ophthalmology and medicine, but also in electronic engineering and nanotechnology. Therefore, these researches should not only make journals specialize in medicine, but the revisions should also include nanotechnology and engineering to make it more accurate. In Figure 2, reports regarding retinal implants that were made by principal countries have been proven evident.

Institutions and universities are making major breakthroughs in the field of retinal implants for more than two decades. In fact, some already have several patents, prototypes, and

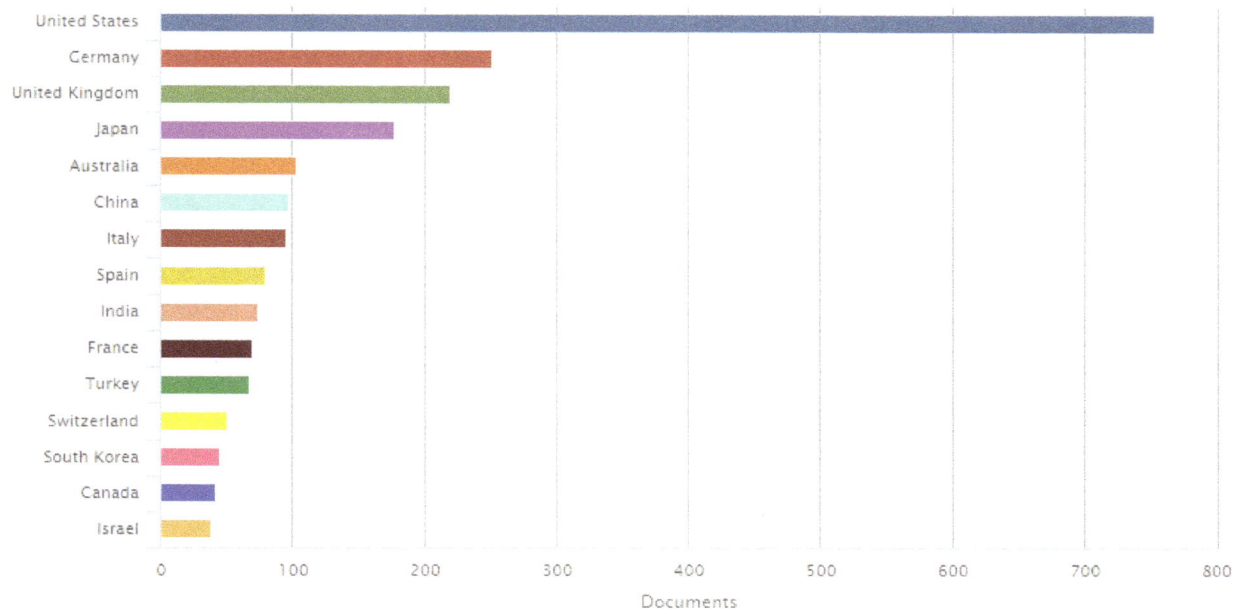

Figure 2. Publications in retinal implants in different countries. Copyright 2015. Elsevier B.V. All right reserved. Scopus is a registered trademark of Elsevier B.V.

experimental models in animals. There is already evidence in humans, which provides a promising future for people with retinitis pigmentosa, which a few years ago would have been considered impossible. See Figure 3 [3].

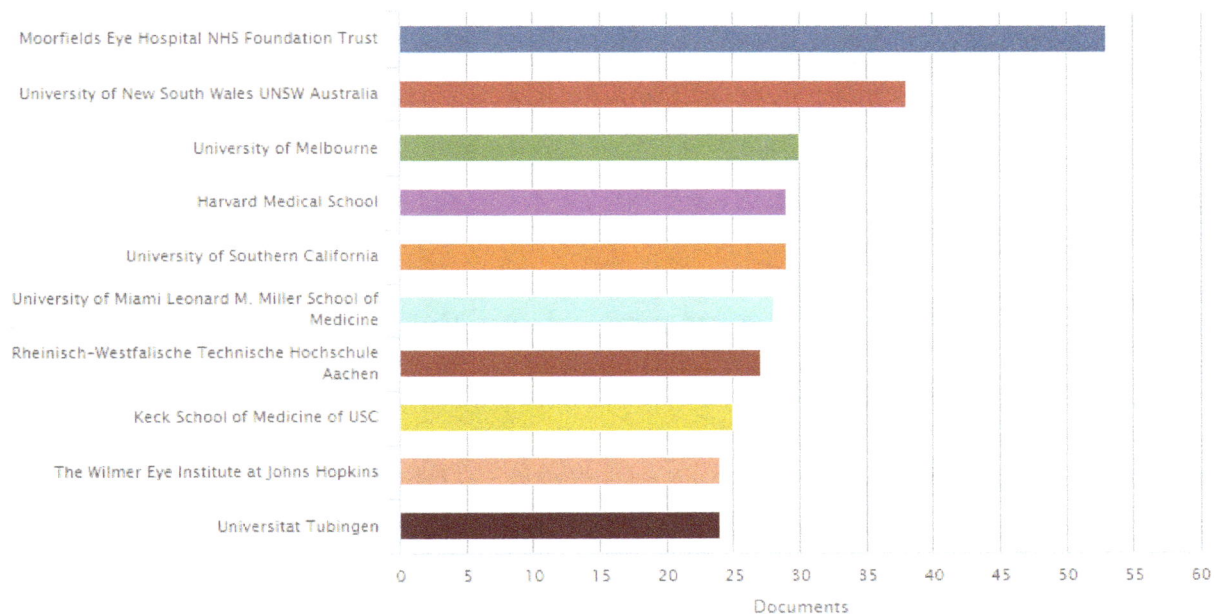

Figure 3. Top Publications in retinal implants for institutes and Universities around the World. Copyright 2015. Elsevier B.V. All right reserved. Scopus is a registered trademark of Elsevier B.V.

4. Types of eye surgery

Today, the classification of eye surgery can be summarized in Figure 4.

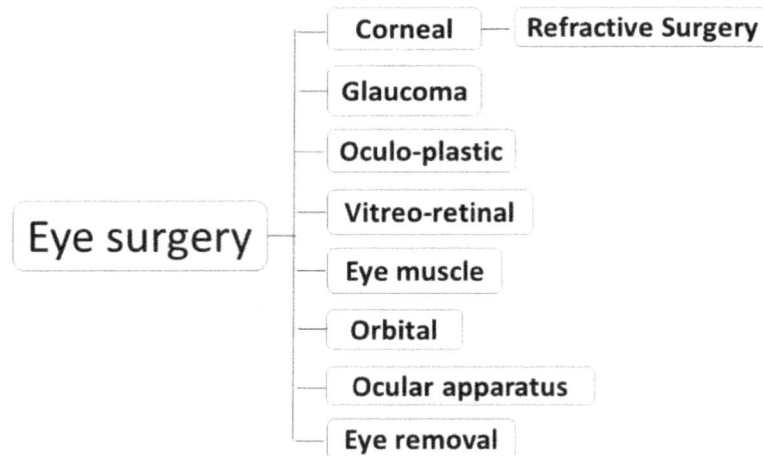

Eye surgery
- Corneal — Refractive Surgery
- Glaucoma
- Oculo-plastic
- Vitreo-retinal
- Eye muscle
- Orbital
- Ocular apparatus
- Eye removal

Figure 4. Classification of the types of eye surgery.

5. Ocular surgical techniques

In the surgery of myopia, astigmatism, and presbyopia, several techniques have improved since the 80s (See figure 5). And recently, a stromal ring technique has been introduced for keratoconus. Due to the shortage of donors for corneas, the stem cell culture and the development of new biopolymers has increased until the creation of several artificial corneas.

6. Corneal surgery

The corneal transplant surgery is useful in the removal and replacement of damaged corneas, replacing it with a clear donor cornea (corneal grafting) in its entirety (penetrating keratoplasty) or in part (lamellar keratoplasty). Another surgical technique is the deep anterior lamellar keratoplasty (remotion of the anterior layers of the central cornea) if the replacement includes posterior cells: endothelia, stroma and Descemets cells (DSEK) or Descemets/endothelium (DMEK).

Boston keratoprosthesis is a synthetic cornea used since 2008 (Boston KPro), which was developed for the Massachusetts Eye and Ear Infirmary. The AlphaCor, a device that contains a peripheral skirt and a transparent central region, is another artificial cornea. The parts connect interpenetrating polymer network made from poly-2-hydoxyethylmethacrylate (pHEMA). Another model is the osteo-odonto-keratoprosthesis, wherein a lamina of the patient's tooth

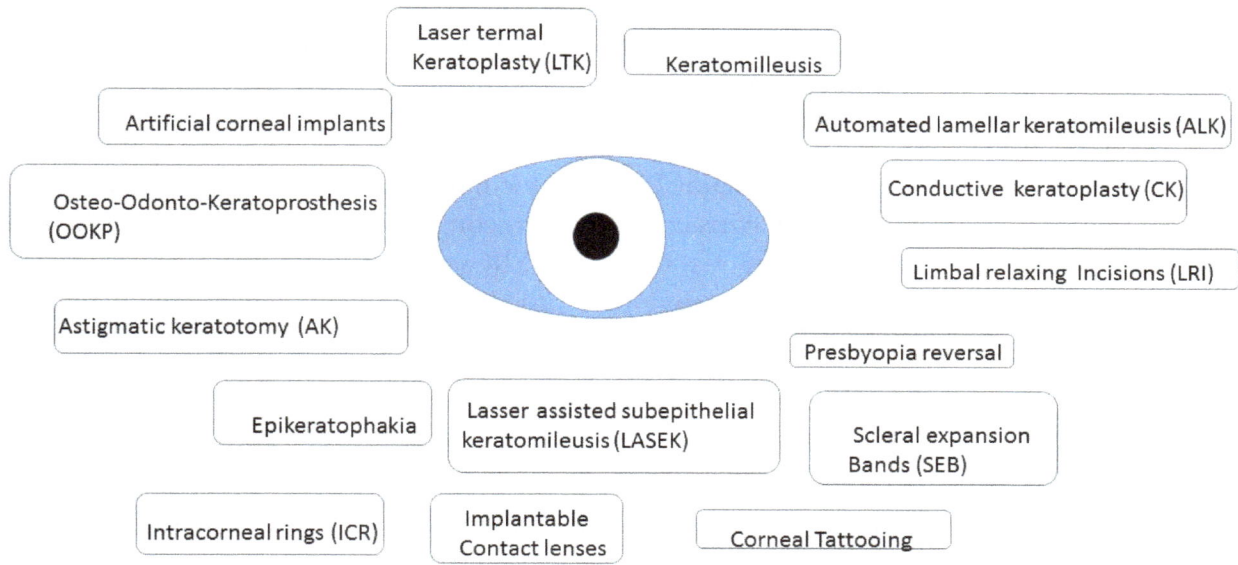

Figure 5. Corneal surgery techniques.

is implanted into the eye using an artificial lens. The porous graphite/PVA hydrogel composite as the skirt of artificial cornea, in the experimental model shows the interconnective porous network. The mechanical properties and water content are similar to nature donor cornea. Water content is another crucial characteristic of hydrogel used as a material for artificial cornea because it will influence the biocompatibility of hydrogel. Experimental studies developed in rabbits in vivo shows that the hydrogel nanocomposite implants of Zn NP were well tolerated in over 3 weeks of study, with no evidence of wound leakage, infection, inflammation, or neovascularization [4].

Corneal cross-linking is a technique used for the treatment of keratoconus. It increases the corneal rigidity by photo polymerization of the stromal collagen fibers with UV light for less than 30 minutes. The standard cross-linking technique, also called Dresden protocol (CXL), requires the removal of the central 9 nm of the corneal epithelium layer followed by 30 minutes of riboflavin administration [5].

In order to make a predictive value pair wing refractive surgery and have a more accurate and useful value for refractive surgery and the stromal rings for keratoconus, sophisticated software have been developed to help surgeons take more precise models before the surgery. Some of them are provided by manufacturers and others have been developed based on sophisticated mathematical models, which are very useful in cases of keratoconus or corneal astigmatism [6].

Nomograms are incisions within the cornea without the need to break the epithelium or Bowman´s, thus avoiding the risk of wound problems and possible overcorrections during refractive surgery. Recently, specialized software products can help surgeons on the different procedures. Some of them are IBRA, Intacs®, and Nomograms (useful for ICRS in keratoconus by the use of a ring base on the type of the cone) [7, 8, 9]. In presbyopia surgery, an optical device as thin as a contact lens is inserted into the cornea to reshape the front surface of the eye in order to improve vision. Corneal inlays are used to improve near vision and reduce the need for reading glasses. This device can be combined with LASIK for nearsightedness, farsightedness, and/or astigmatism.

This procedure is less invasive than phakic IOL (intraocular lenses placed deeper in the eye). So, with the corneal inlays for vision correction, eye surgeons may sometimes be able to avoid complications associated with procedures, such as LASIK and PRK, because no corneal tissue is removed. The Kamra Corneal Inlay, previously called ACI 7000, for presbyopia is now in clinical trials. The device in inserted in a thin flap in the center of the cornea. The flap is then replaced over the inlay to hold it in place in a process of 15 minutes [10].

Its innovation holds a promise to replace reading glasses with good near vision in the near future. The characteristics of Kamra are described as follows: 3.8 millimeters in diameter, 10 microns thick, made of an opaque biocompatible polymer (Kynar), and a thermoplastic material that softens in heat and hardens in cooler conditions.

Corneal inlays and onlays are also called keratophakia. They are implants placed in the corneal stroma for the correction of presbyopia. The procedure is done under topical anesthesia and the implant is done monocularly in the non-dominant eye as a stromal pocket or under the flaps created by the microkeratome or by the femtosecond laser. See Figure 6.

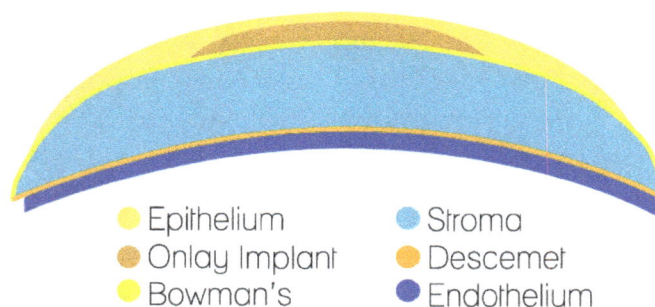

Epithelium   Stroma
Onlay Implant   Descemet
Bowman's   Endothelium

Figure 6. Position of the corneal onlay implants.

Other innovations for these techniques have been developed for researchers in Mexico, who are working on Raindrop near Vision Inlay (ReVision Optics) with some variation on diameters, thickness, and biomaterials.

This inlay is placed in the cornea under a LASIK-style flap. When in position, the inlay changes the curvature of the cornea so the front of the eye acts much like a multifocal contact lens. The other alternative is the Flexivue Microlens (Presbia Cooperatief U.A., Amsterdam), which uses a laser and creates a tiny pocket just below the eye's surface. Currently, it requires developing the instrument to insert the microlens in the pocket that is sealed to hold the lens, and a hydrophilic polymer is irrigated during surgery with a highly moisturizing substance. The synthetic intraocular lens replaces the natural lens during cataract surgery. Its characteristics are as follows: 3 mm in diameter and 20 microns thick at the edges [11].

7. 3D Models for training and surgery

7.1. Glaucoma

Some helpful preoperative aids recently included for prior surgery are the 3D models. These must be used to investigate the pressure drop on the localization of the main resistance to aqueous egress during iridectomy or trabeculectomy surgery. Some of these are the modeling of the eye drainage using the computational fluid dynamics (CFD) and the eye drainage system devices (GDD). To provide a 3D CFD prototype of the eye, the basis is the anatomy of a real human eye. Some models are based on stacks of microphotographs from human eye slides from which digital processing of the images of the eye structure and 3D reconstruction of the model are performed. The simulations of the distribution of pressure and the flow velocity in the model of a healthy eye bring results comparable to physiology references. Mimicking glaucoma conditions, most likely the real eye, led to an increase of the IOP from normal range, which went down to lower values after a filtering procedure. With this, a computer assisted design (CAD) model of the device is inserted in the 3D eye through the DC and the trabecular meshwork of the anterior chamber angle, parallel to the plane of the iris [12].

7.2. Cataract surgery

A simulation, very similar to the real environment, has been implemented, so the training for the surgeon is more secure. It is also in real-time as a virtual simulator with a control position tracking in a stereoscopic display mounted on a head, with a video, audio, and haptic interface in virtual reality. A real environment has been simulated that is created electronically in a controlled and protected environment where the surgeon can learn, practice, and improve their skills for surgery in a safe environment [13].

SensAble Phantom Omni [T.M] is equipped with a device that controls virtual surgical instruments and feeds the skills of the surgeon, allowing six degrees of freedom tracking, three of which are important in human-machine interface for simulation. A haptic interface is designed to identify the types of surgical operations, such as cutting, grasping, pushing, emulsion, and calculated reaction force, and allows modeling the deformation of the mesh fabric, such as an eye model. The cyanoacrylate polymerizes as soon as it touches something like water and aqueous or saline solution. Fibrin glue is also another sealant that is also used for pterygium with conjunctival auto-grafts and secures amniotic membrane tissue in pterygium surgery. Sealants made of polyethylene glycol hydrogel are used for sealing corneal incisions and implantation in the IOL [14].

8. 3D Bioprinting

3D printing, better known as bioprinting, has been widely accepted in the health industry. This was initially developed to print 3D process designs in the gastronomy industry. Later on, it has become one alternative medicine for organ replacement. Printing with organs like heart, liver, kidney, replacement hip bones, and maxillofacial trachea has become an alternative in association with research on stem cells to regenerate tissue. Eye level attempts have been cast for 3D modeling and future impressions of the eyeball for cosmetic purposes in people requiring ocular prostheses turned what was previously artisanal towards a more precise subsequent enucleation process. This improves the aesthetic value and lowers the probability of infection that occurs in these tissues due to poor hygiene because there is no need to frequently remove it for cleaning purposes [15].

This process consists of the printing, layer by layer, on a 3D printer using stable biological materials applied in tissue engineering. Very few materials, which fulfill the requirements for bioprinting as well as provide adequate properties for cell encapsulation during and after the printing process, are available. Some of the materials that are similar to the contact lens hydrogel composite or include alginate and gelatin precursors were tuned with different concentrations of hydroxyapatite (HA) and were characterized in terms of rheology, which is the swelling behavior and mechanical properties used to assess the versatility of the system properties [16].

9. Development on visual implants

The LIS-CEA laboratory in France has been studying retinal implants from nanomaterials and nanodiamonds. By means of the implementation of memristors and digital technology, electronic devices that respond to Moore's Law (processing speed, memory capacity, and number of pixels) inspired the creation of cardiac pacemakers and created an intelligent flash. This concept was introduced by Leon O. Chua and was developed as a model of neural networks, the biomimetic model of the retina, where they expected to even send 3D signals. [17].

A project was undertaken wherein other technologies using silicon microchips as a "wafer" to create a biological and electronic device in the form of functional circuits that interact with live cells and shows a promise for the present and future cells. The construction of the small three-dimensional models of the human organs can be used to treat and replace costly and time-consuming animal studies that currently hamper the development of drugs. Furthermore, these micro-electromechanical systems (MEMS) allow testing in cell cultures without using a full tissue. A lab-on-a-chip enables the replication of tissue samples [18].

FDA approved a project of more than 15 years which comprised an interdisciplinary group of researchers. The retinal prosthesis was created: Second Sight Argus II, with funding from the National Eye Institute. It consists of a camera that captures images via implanted electrodes that stimulate cells in the retina, producing a light on the patient's visual field. This camera mounted on a pair of eyeglasses wirelessly (with 60 electrodes and hoping to increase it to 1500), has an array of microelectrodes and is mounted on a miniature camera on a pair of glasses that act as a sensitive photodiode light. The camcorder captures a portion of the visual field and transmits the information to the VPU. The device is already being used in patients with retinitis pigmentosa [19].

Traditionally, the aesthetics of the manufacturing and fitting of ocular prostheses are acceptable and responds efficiently in improving the patient's confidence and physical and psychological well-being, therefore, helps to improve their social acceptance and quality of life. Recently, the introduction of visual implants is a different alternative designed to transmit electronical signals from the retina to the brain. According to the surgical technique and position, they are inserted or transplanted into the body and tend to be used as a therapeutic instrument for visual rehabilitation. The artificial stimulation to the visual pathway allows the brain to recognize the electric signal as light. New electronical materials useful for the fabrication of these devices have been developed in the recent years. An ocular prosthesis helps the patient psychologically and improves confidence, but doesn't have a visual function. Different techniques are available to fabricate a custom ocular prosthesis. In contrast, visual implants are currently being developed as an innovation to restore nerve impulses between the eyeball and the cerebral cortex, linking transdisciplinary efforts, electronic engineers, and ophthalmologists worldwide working to develop the bionic eye. The researchers are focused to allow and improve the perception of spots of light and high contrast edges by means of the devices' stimulator as electrodes or optogenetics transducers.

See Figure 6 [20].

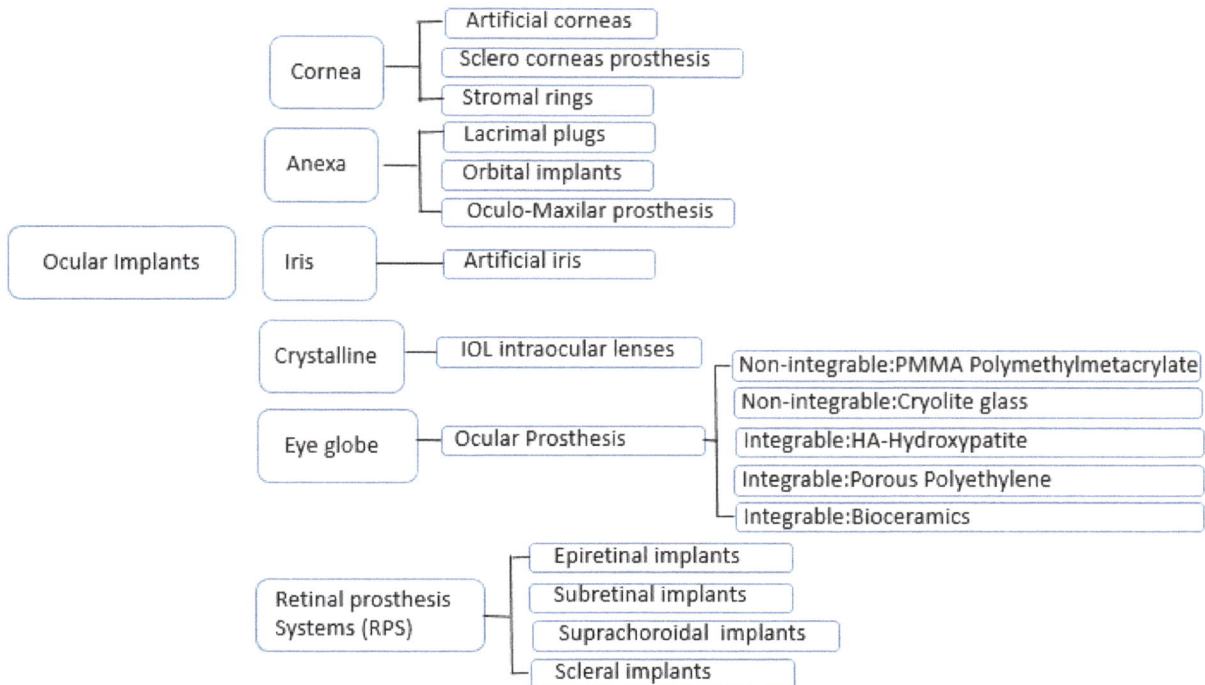

Figure 7. Classification of Ocular implants. Durán, P. Diaz, M, Plaza, J. Journal of ocular diseases and therapeutics. 2 N. 1, 2014.

Ocular prostheses were made and are still fabricated in inhert and non-integrable materials, such as polymethylmetacrylate (PMMA) and cryolite glass. But these days, integrable materials for anophthalmic cavities, such as a gel from cellulose produced by Zoogloea sp.

porous polyethylene dental biomaterial composites and graphene among others, are implemented as materials for the heart, eye and other organs implants due to their characteristics in improving biological compatibility to be more resistant, to reduce allergies, and improve durability. The future development of the ocular prostheses is focused on the impression of digital measurements, 3D modeling software, and the digital impression of the iris [21].

Many implants are being studied around the world. Some patents and other humans have been implanted to help in visual rehabilitation. Some of these examples are divided into two categories according to design or operations principles, some use an external camera and image processing drive implanted electrodes. Another example is the use of 1500 small units in microphotodiode arrays (MPA by Retina Implant AG) and Stanford retinal prosthesis. Some required external energy to drive the stimulators, while others are wireless. The Stanford array projects a high intensity infrared image on the implanted photocells and generates a sufficient current to excite the secondary neurons. In addition, the classification must be made according to the implant site e.g., in the inner retinal (epiretinal) or outer (subretinal) retinal surface; if the implant is inserted below the choroid plexus (suprachoroidal) or if the implantation take place outside the sclera (episcleral) [22, 23, 24].

Before the production of visual implants, many studies should be performed to verify the noise pattern, the extraction processing of the temporal space, monitoring to check the quality of the image, the spatial resolution, the circuit architecture, and advanced intelligent functions.

The future smart 3D image sensor architectures will most probably consist of a sensor layer at the top and various processing layers below. Each layer will be organized into locally connected cellular arrays with additional global communication/operation mechanisms. Layers will be vertically interconnected using bi-directional parallel channels implemented by through-silicon-vias (TSVs). Images at different scales and abstract information about salient points and features will be transmitted top-down across the stack, while commands will be transmitted bottom-up to support adaptation.

10. Optical Coherence Tomography (OCT) in surgery

The OCT has revolutionized the clinical management of ophthalmic diseases and promises to be of great help in the surgical rooms. The Prospective Intraoperative and Perioperative Ophthalmic Imaging with Optical Coherence Tomography (PIONEER), a single site multi-surgeon prospective is incorporating the OCT to the surgical room because of feasibility, safety, and utility. This study is performed by the Cleveland Clinic. The variables including past ocular history, procedure type, preoperative diagnosis, techniques, and number of imaging sessions are recorded one day before surgery. The structured study follow-up is done after the surgery [25].

The protocol managing for them is next. Disease-specific or procedure-specific imaging protocols (eg. scan type, pattern, density, size, orientation) were outlined for anterior and posterior segment applications. Anterior segment imaging included a 12mm^3, 12mm volumetric cube scan at 0 degree orientation. Posterior segment imaging included a 10 mm^3, 10 mm volumetric cube with 100 B-scans per volume at both 0 and 90 degrees, a 5 - 3 10mm volumetric cube with 7 B-scans per frame for averaging, a total of 175 B-scans per volume at both 0 and 90 degrees, and a 10 mm radial scan with 100 B-scans per volume. The surgeons were provided with guidance for surgical milestones to consider for imaging (e.g., pre-incision, following membrane peeling, following graft placement), but the specific imaging sessions were at the surgeon's discretion. When possible in vitreoretinal cases, scan sequences were obtained in the operating room prior to any surgical manipulation of the area of interest. Following various surgical milestones, scan sequences were performed to allow for comparative data and change analysis. A "scan" was defined as a single set of images. A "scan session" was defined as a series of scans obtained during a single pause during surgery. Typically, multiple scan sessions were often performed during the surgical procedures. A specific surgical procedure (e.g., Membrane peeling, lamellar keratoplasty) intraoperative OCT feedback form was included as part of the study protocol. This form included questions regarding the impact of the intraoperative OCT on surgical decision making and on how intraoperative OCT may have impacted the understanding of the surgical disease of interest. OCT provides rapid testing that reduces costs, time, and enhances quality care for surgeons and patients [26].

11. Further research

Future research of new innovations in visual implants improves existing research for best results. The early implementation of refractive surgery and cataract surgery is recalled, however, it is important that the increase of that research is conducted in global scientific communities where you can monitor patients and have access to people with visual impairment that requires the surgery. High costs should be borne by health systems, according to the laws of each country, so that they can be taken advantage by the patients who need them. Some of the challenges that are presented in eye health are the cost of the technology transfer, more high-level training in surgical procedures, and the establishment of protocols according to the clinical findings. Just as eye surgery has been the pioneer in the world among many technological advancements, it becomes a possible reality in the near future to restore vision for visual rehabilitation and to provide a better quality of life for visually impaired patients.

Likewise, due to the interaction of the new sciences, ophthalmologists around the world should have comprehensive training from his clinical practice in various branches of medicine, biomedical engineering and electronics, and nanotechnology. Team groups with different point of views must be formed to answer the needs of patients, such as applying science to the clinic, establishing protocols to prevent errors, and improve processes in eye surgery and thus, optimizing costs, human resources and effectiveness for patients. All these innovations must be reimbursed by health insurance systems around the world.

So that these advancements reach patients, there should be access to global insurance to cover the population that needs them. Germany and the United States are already doing this. However, in underdeveloped countries, this possibility does not even exist and is yet to be built.

The truth is that in the near future, these new surgeries may have results that help reduce blindness, improve the coverage and quality of life for patients with myopia, astigmatism, presbyopia, cataracts, and retinitis pigmentosa among others. The inclusion of contact lenses has always been considered as one of the most important innovations for mankind. But this technology is linked to new projects and has developed new biopolymers. The challenge for innovators and surgeons in the next decades is the immersion with electronic chips. The accuracy of current studies is required and must be taken advantage by the academic community for the scientific needs and reading of the general population.

Another important area in future work on education to transfer this technology and provide updates with experts and developers for the patients' safety, must be worked in partnership with the different industries and academia.

12. Conclusion

Eye surgery is not only considered a pioneer in the world by technological advancements, but evidence also shows that it has been and will continue to be important to combat blindness in the world. Among the most significant advancements are visual implants, artificial corneas, new biopolymers, and the inclusion of nanotechnology in operating rooms where other major global challenges will come from.

The challenge of new visual innovation includes multiple fields that must continue to be improved for these new global developments in refractive surgery, ocular prosthesis, and visual implants. In order to make these advancements accessible to patients, it is required to improve the transfer of technology and improve the training of surgeons around the world. The following points must also be taken into consideration:

1. Eye surgery research: strengthening global researchers' mobility and internships among researchers of visual health-electronical engineering groups around the world to be training in transdisciplinary teams about the new surgical technique and developments in electronic engineering and their applications to visual health. It must include developments for other healthcare artifacts.

2. Financial resources: search financial resources from government and public and private entities to develop new technology transfer policies.

3. Database creation for target population in visual implants or visual rehabilitation: the creation of a global database of possible patients that can benefit from these innovations should be a priority in each country and will make us plan for monitoring, check the progress in new implanted patients, verify the recovery rates, and design a project of the improvement thereof.

4. Challenge for Institutional Review Boards (IRB committees) of academic institutions: The Institutional Review

5. Boards of universities around the world should construct and share global protocols about new technology surgery: to take care of the visual implants, fill up the informed consent

in the use of these new innovations, provide mechanisms for timely and appropriate communication to users, investors, and inventors, and report the cost - benefits of these new alternatives.

6. Marketing: The other challenge is the distribution channels. A highly qualified medical and rehabilitation staff is required after the implantation: a team of psychological support, visual rehabilitators, and low vision experts around the world. Most importantly, family support is key for a successful visual recovery. In the case of ocular prosthesis, the personal cleaning regime requires periodic professional care. Some authors have proposed the three phase model according to the discharge associated with prosthetic eye wear. In the initial period, the freshly polished prosthesis set the homeostasis in the first phase as surface deposits are removed is more comfortable and safer. However, you can make an increased likelihood of harm when continued wear, that´s is the reason to think in recovers such as nanofilms or new biopolymer can reduce the deposits another way is the traditional surface polish. There is not too much published literature about maintenance care of visual prosthesis, electrodes and microarrays.

The new research for eye surgery is focused on the development of artificial organs, ocular prosthesis, and the inclusion of new biomaterials as graphene or nanocoatings against biofilm and microorganisms. This creates digitalized prototypes and is customized for each patient, using new technology and working with 3D printing organs. Some advancements have been developed in the United Kingdom, in partnership with Fripp Design and Research and Manchester Metropolitan University, using the Spectrum Z-Corp 510 3D printer. The main reason for inclusion of graphene as an ocular biomaterial is because this material serves as a photovoltaic semiconductor, which is unlike the metal or silicon-based materials used until now for such biotechnological interfaces. The graphene is soft, light, flexible and highly biocompatible. Naturally, new biomaterials and neuro-implants is the challenge for visual care for sensitivity to visible light. It uses photovoltaic material and does not require an external electrical source to function.

Nomenclature

AK: Astigmatic Keratoplasty

ALK: Automated lamellar keratomileusis

BANG: Bits, Atoms, Neurons, and Genes.

CK: Conductive keratoplasty

GNR: Genetics, Nanotechnology and Robotics.

GRIN: Genetic, Robotic, Information, and Nanotechnology.

ICR: Intracorneal rings.

LRI: Limbal relaxing keratoplasty

LTK: Laser termal keratoplasty

NBIC: Nanotechnology, Biotechnology, Information technology and Cognitive science.

OOKP: Osteo-Odonto-Keratoprosthesis

LASEK: Lasser assisted subepithelial keratomileusis

OCT: Optical Coherence Tomography

PIONEER: Prospective Intraoperative and Perioperative Ophthalmic Imaging With Optical Coherence Tomography

SEB: scleral expansion bands

Acknowledgements

Thanks to Veronica Barbudo Duran, Graphic designer, for her graphics and design contributions for the chapter.

Author details

Patricia Durán Ospina[1*], Mayra Catalina Cáceres Díaz[1] and Sabrina Lara[2]

*Address all correspondence to: pduran@areandina.edu.co

1 Visual Research Group Fundación Universitaria del Área Andina, Pereira, Colombia

2 Universidad Nacional de Villa María, Córdoba, Argentina

References

[1] Durán, P. Are nanotechnology and robotics alternatives for therapeutic and theragnostic ophthalmic applications technologies for eye care services. Journal of ocular diseases and therapeutics. Savvy Science. Pg 24 – 32. DOI: http://dx.doi.org/10.12974/2309-6136.2013.01.01.6 Download at: http://savvysciencepublisher.com/downloads/jodtv1n1a6/.

[2] Bainoa, F. Pereroa, F., Ferrarisa, S., Miola, M. Balagnaa, C., Vernéa,E. Chiara Vitale-Brovaronea, Coggiolac, A. Dolcinoc, D., Ferrarisa. M. Biomaterials for orbital implants and ocular prostheses: Overview and future prospects. Acta Biomaterialia. Volume 10, Issue 3, March 2014, Pages 1064–1087. http://dx.doi.org/10.1016/j.actbio.2013.12.014.

[3] Scopus database. Elsevier. Analyzer. Consult date. January 2015.

[4] Zhang Q., Su Q., Chan-Park M.B. et al. Development of high refractive ZnS/PVP/PDMAA hydrogel nanocomposites for artificial cornea implants. Acta Biomaterialia 10 (2014) 1167–1176.

[5] Romppainen, T.; Bachmann, L. M.; Kaufmann, C.; Kniestedt, C.; Mrochen, M.; Thiel, M. A. (1 December 2007). "Effect of Riboflavin-UVA Induced Collagen Cross-linking on Intraocular Pressure Measurement". Investigative Ophthalmology & Visual Science. pp. 5494–5498. doi:10.1167/iovs.06-1479.

[6] Pine, K., Sloan,B., Jacobs.R. A proposed model of the response of the anophthalmic socket to prosthetic eyewear and its application to the management of mucoid discharge. Department of Optometry and Vision Science, New Zealand National Eye Centre, The University of Auckland, New Zealand. Medical Hypotheses - August 2013 (Vol. 81, Issue 2, Pages 300-305, DOI: 10.1016/j.mehy.2013.04.024).

[7] Shetty,R. D'Souza, S. et al. Decision making nomogram for intrastromal corneal ring segments in keratoconus. Indian J Ophthalmol 2014. Jan 4; 62(1): 23–28.doi: 10.4103/0301-4738.126170.

[8] Gortzak, R., Willem Jan. et al. Advanced personalized nomogram for myopic laser surgery: First 100 eyes. http://www.retina.nl/downloads/jaarcijfers_november_2008.pdf. Consulted on January 5 2014.

[9] IBRA Software. https://www.zubisoft.com/http/overview.php. Consulted on January 5 2014.

[10] Güell J., Arrada O. Intracorneal Inlays – Special Focus on the Raindrop Ophthalmic Review, 2014;7(2):123–30 http://www.touchophthalmology.com/articles/intracorneal-inlays-special-focus-raindrop-0. Consulted January 2015.

[11] Presbia Flexivue Microlens procedure. http://presbia.com/surgery/index.php. Consulted January 2015.

[12] Villamarin, A., Roy, S., H. Reda et al. 3D simulation of the aqueous flow in the human eye. Medical Engineering & Physics 34 (2012) 1462– 1470. DOI: http://dx.doi.org/10.1016/j.medengphy.2012.02.007.

[13] Kiang Ch., Sundaraja, K., Sulaiman, N. Virtual reality simulator for phacoemulsification cataract surgery education and training. Procedia Computer Science 18 (2013) 742 – 748.

[14] Agarwal A, Jacob S, Kumar DA, Narasimhan S. Handshake technique for glued intrascleral haptic fixation of a posterior chamber intraocular lens. J Cataract Refract Surg. 2013; 39:3:317-22: http://www.reviewofophthalmology.com/content/d/technology_update/c/49801/#sthash.qGdheAxS.dpuf

[15]   Artopoulou, I. Montgomery, P. Wesley, JP. Lemon, J. Digital imaging in the fabrication of ocular prostheses *The Journal of Prosthetic Dentistry, Volume 95, Issue 4, April 2006, Pages 327-330.* http://dx.doi.org/10.1016/j.prosdent.2006.01.018.

[16]   Conesse, M. Bioprinting: A further step to effective regenerative medicine and Tissue Engineering.http://omicsgroup.org/journals/bioprinting-a-further-step-to-effective-regenerative-medicine-and-tissue-engineering-2169-0111.1000e112.pdf.   Consulted January 2015.

[17]   Bengonzo P. Diamond to Retina Artificial Micro-Interface Structures. In France 2010; pp. 1-10. Available on http://cordis.europa.eu/documents/documentlibrary/123542961EN6.pdf. (Accessed March 2013).

[18]   Bhisitkul RB, Keller CG. Development of Microelectromechanical Systems (MEMS) forceps for intraocular surgery. Br J Ophthalmol 2005; 89 (12): 1586-8. http://dx.doi.org/10.1136/bjo.2005.075853.

[19]   Da Cruz L, Coley BF, Dorn J, Merlini F, Filley E, Christopher P, et al. The Argus II epiretinal prosthesis system allows letter and word reading and long-term function in patients with profound vision loss. Br. J Ophthalmol 2013;97(5): 632- 6.http://dx.doi.org/10.1136/bjophthalmol-2012-301525.

[20]   Durán, P. Cáceres, M. Plaza, J. A Review in Innovation in Ocular Prostheses and Visual Implants: New Biomaterials and Neuro-Implants is the Challenge for the Visual Care. Journal of ocular diseases and therapeutics. DOI:0020http://dx.doi.org/10.12974/2309-6136.2014.02.01.3 Download at http://savvysciencepublisher.com/downloads/jodtv2n1a3/.

[21]   Cordeiro-Barbosa Francisco de Assis, Aguiar José Lamartine de Andrade, Lira Mariana Montenegro de Melo, Pontes Filho Nicodemos Teles de, Bernardino-Araújo Sidcley. Use of a gel biopolymer for the treatment of eviscerated eyes: experimental model in rabbits. Arq. Bras. Oftalmol. [serial on the Internet]. 2012. Aug [cited 2013 Dec 26] ; 75(4): 267-272. Available from: http://dx.doi.org/10.1590/S0004-27492012000400010

[22]   Chen J, Patil S, Seal S, McGinnis JF. Rare earth nanoparticles prevent retinal degeneration induced by intracellular peroxides. Nature Nanotechnology. 2006 Nov;1(2): 142-50.

[23]   Chow, A.Y.Chow, V.Y. Artificial retina device with stimulating and ground return electrodes disposed on opposite sides of the neuroretina and method of attachment. https://www.google.de/patents/US8306626. 2012.

[24]   Ehlers JP, Tao YK, Farsiu S, Maldonado R, Izatt JA, Toth CA. Integration of a spectral domain optical coherence tomography system into a surgical microscope for intraoperative imaging. Invest Ophthalmol Vis Sci. 2011 May 16;52(6):3153-9. doi: 10.1167/iovs.10-6720.

[25] Ehlers, J. Dupps, W. et al. The Prospective Intraoperative and Perioperative Ophthalmic Imaging with Optical Coherence Tomography (PIONEER) Study: 2-Year Results. Am J Ophthalmol. 2014 Nov;158(5):999-1007. doi: 10.1016/j.ajo.2014.07.034. Epub 2014 Jul 29.

[26] Tao YK, Srivastava SK, Ehlers JP. Microscope-integrated intraoperative OCT with electrically tunable focus and heads-up display for imaging of ophthalmic surgical maneuvers. Biomed Opt Express 2014; 5(6):1877–1885. doi: 10.1364/BOE.5.001877

6

Minimally Invasive Sutureless Day Case Vitrectomy Surgery for Retinal Detachments, Floaters, Macular Holes and Epiretinal Membranes

Lik Thai Lim and Ahmed El-Amir

Abstract

This chapter takes an ophthalmologist through vitreo-retinal (VR) surgery from the beginning to the end, using a case-based approach to highlight the skills required, lessons learnt from and pit-falls to avoid in VR surgery. This is especially useful to those who are new and intermediate VR surgeons.

The case represents the common conditions requiring VR surgery, so that the reader can get exposure from the common cases, ranging from hot cases like retinal detachment, to cold cases like macular hole surgery and epiretinal membrane peel, and important cases like diabetic VR cases and trauma cases.

Keywords: Vitreo-retinal, surgery, retina, vitreous

1. Introduction

Vitreoretinal (VR) surgery is an ever-changing speciality with newer and more effective instruments and equipments being introduced constantly over time. Long gone were the days when 20 gauge vitrectomy was first introduced. We now have 23, 25 and 27 gauge systems with improved duty cycles and cut rates aiding the safety and results for patients [1, 2, 3]. Although the instruments maybe updated from time to time, certain basic VR surgical techniques remain core to any VR operation.

This chapter is aimed at taking the reader from the basics in learning and performing VR surgery, touching on the main basic principles and building on with surgical pearls, some of which are not found in standard VR textbooks. Whenever possible, there will be a link provided to access short video clips to reiterate the techniques and concepts discussed, making this an interactive chapter. As such, the beginner and the intermediate-level surgeons will benefit from this chapter, with points for the advanced surgeon.

As there are many different models and types of vitrectomy machines, the discussion in this chapter will will focus on the concepts and techniques and parameters common to all machines. It is expected that the reader is familiar with the commonly used instruments for VR surgery.

This chapter is not meant to substitute a standard VR surgery textbook but merely an informative supplementary chapter focussing on practical techniques. The chapter is arranged in a gradual way of introducing VR surgery starting from simple cases through to more complex cases, with clinical pearls and discussion of techniques and learning points for each case. The approach to this chapter shall be case based. It is assumed that the readers would be familiar and well versed in the basic anatomy, physiology, and pathology of the eye. However, relevant consideration in basic sciences will be reiterated to highlighting surgical principles and concepts in a more memorable way. Each case is presented with learning points and is itemised for easier read and revision.

It is hoped that the techniques and approach to VR surgery discussed in this chapter will allow the reader to adopt a flexible and appropriate combination of techniques and approaches to meet the individual surgical requirements that each case merits, in a safe and controlled manner, given that VR can be an unforgiving subspecialty if not performed expertly.

2. General considerations for the new VR surgeons

It is important to ensure that the patient is comfortable and the cornea is parallel with the floor. The surgeons position should also be comfortable.

Please note that the anterior vitreous base is 1 mm in front of the recti insertion, and the posterior vitreous base is 3–5 mm behind the recti insertion. The ora is at the insertion line of all the recti except for the superior rectus, which is 1 mm in front of the superior rectus insertion.

Setting up of the three port pars plana vitrectomy (PPV) is a crucial start of the surgery, and each step needs to be meticulously performed. The positions of the three trocars are in the inferotemporal quadrant, superotemporal quadrant, and superonasal quadrant. Each trocar should be placed at an appropriate distance from the limbus, with 4 mm away from the limbus if the patient is phakic and 3.5 mm away for pseudophakic patients.

Since most centres have moved towards small gauge ports [4, 5, 6], with many surgeons preferring the sutureless transconjunctival sclerostomies, the technique to perform the sclerostomies needs to be mentioned here. The trocar needs to be inserted obliquely (approximately 45°) till midscleral depth, before the trocar is reposition perpendicular to the sclera to complete the sclerostomy incision [7, 8]. This will result in a shelved wound for better self-sealing (similar idea as the main phacoemulsification corneal stepped incision for self-sealing effect). Recent evidence from endosurgical imaging techniques presented at the American Academy of Ophthalmology meeting 2015 shows that a 2-step insertion technique can cause trauma and 'stretch' to the pars plana possibly increasing a risk of an entry-site tear or haemorrhage. Therefore some experts recommend a 1-step insertion technique. Clinical experience suggests that this risk is low (1 in 300 cases).

The infusion line needs to be checked and allowed to flow before insertion to allow air bubbles to be expelled before connecting to the inferotemporal trocar. Before switching on the infusion, check to make sure that the infusion cannula is in the vitreous cavity and not anywhere else, pointing towards the centre of the vitreous cavity. Then the infusion is switched on.Remember to switch on the inverter on the operating microscope to facilitate the correct view of the retina. Some systems such as the Carl Zeiss system do this automatically. Others will invert manually by a hand switch or a foot switch.

There are also many different types of binocular indirect ophthalmic microscope viewing system (BIOM system) for viewing the retina for VR surgery. Regardless of the system used, the basic principle for retinal surgical work (apart from macula work) requires a wide view. In this situation, the microscope is zoomed out to the maximum, and the BIOM lens is adjusted until a clear focus is obtained. Then the microscope is lowered until a wide clear view is obtained which involves the BIOM lens being a few millimetres away from the cornea.

The general principle of vitrectomy is to surgically remove most of the vitreous, to allow the surgeon to do whatever retinal work that is required. With the vitreous cavity illuminated (either with handheld light pipe or chandelier light), the vitrector is introduced into one of the trocars, and core vitrectomy is performed at the centre of the vitreous cavity. Then posterior vitreous detachment (PVD) is checked. If it is absent, then a PVD should be induced. If PVD is present, then peripheral shave of the vitreous should be performed after core vitrectomy. The peripheral shave is a dynamic process requiring constant eye–hand–feet coordination (moving the X–Y shift of the microscope foot pedal), moving around the vitreous base as the vitrectomy is going on. This will allow for optimal visualisation of the area being vitrectomised.

The technique to get a good thin shave of the vitreous is to tilt the eye as much as possible towards the vitrector with the vitrector being placed at the edge of the optimal peripheral retinal view. The peripheral shave is performed systematically. The vitrector is placed at the edge of the fundal view in order to get as close a shave as possible, with the vitrector being placed at a clock hour for approximately 10–15 seconds to ensure a good shave before moving on to the next clock hour. Especially for phakic eyes, it is important to not cross the midline to avoid lenticular touch. Ensure the port of the vitrector is always facing away from the retina to avoid retinal incarceration.

The induction of PVD requires certain basic consideration, although there are different approaches (varying among surgeons). As the vitreous is attached at its strongest point in the ora serrata and the optic disc, and the induction of PVD is done near the optic disc, the vitrector should be switched to aspiration only and directed towards the optic disc. By increasing the aspiration rate, the vitrector cutter orifice is swirled hovering above the optic disc in a slow methodical manner to capture the bulk of vitreous body before it is pulled tangentially away to the midperiphery of the retina, avoiding the macula and major arcades. Once reaching midperiphery, then the surgeon can switch to cut to release the tip of the vitrector from vitreous. The process is repeated until a definite PVD is obtained. Once PVD is induced, then the surgeon can continue with the peripheral shave as described above.

Now that we have reviewed the basic steps of vitrectomy, we are now going to discuss more techniques and methods tried and tested for a more effective and safer VR surgery through a case based discussion format.

3. VR cases for further practical learning points

Case 1: Macula-off retinal detachment (RD) with multiple holes in 3–4 quadrants in a phakic patient, with posterior vitreous detachment (PVD) positive

In this first case of RD, we take the reader through the steps in RD repair (although there may be slight variations among different surgeons). Subsequent points will just highlight learning points for that particular case, with the assumption that the reader would have been familiar with the surgical steps in VR surgery, as discussed in the introduction section.

1. Three port pars plana vitrectomy (PPV)

2. Core vitrectomy followed by the induction of PVD if not present. Otherwise, continue with core vitrectomy followed by peripheral vitreous shave.

3. Do not cross midline to avoid lenticular touch in phakic eyes.

4. Careful vitrectomy is done near to the retinal break with minimal vacuum and vitrector cut rate to relieve traction while minimising iatrogenic breaks or widening the existing break. This can be done by increasing the cut rate and reducing the aspiration rate when vitrectomising near the break.

5. After the vitrectomy is performed, assess if the retinal break causing the RD is vital. By touching the retina break area, the surgeon can then assess for vitreous traction.

6. Steps 5 and 6 can be repeated until all traction is relieved.

7. Then indent the sclera (e.g., by using a squint hook) to check for other breaks all round, after the irrigation pressure is reduced (e.g., 10 mmHg).

8. Cryotherapy of the break/s can be done in either saline (as long as detached retina layer can be indented by the cryoprobe to be in opposition with the choroid layer) or air (with or without diathermy marking). Diathermy around the area of break/s especially small breaks will make it easier for the surgeon to identify break/s for cryoretinopexy. Care needs to be taken so that the area of lesion will not be over treated with cryotherapy. This can lead to thinning of sclera, sclera necrosis, and scleritis. In our practice, a definite whitening of the area being cryoed is considered as adequate cryoreaction.

9. Backflush (flute) is used to drain subretinal fluid (SRF) from near the break in an accessible area. The flute cannula should be placed in a position hovering above the break so that the SRF can be drained, and at the same time not catching on the retina, being a passive aspiration instrument.

10. Heavy liquid (HL) (e.g., perfluorodecalin) is used to flatten retina. The advantages of this are multifold. First, it helps stabilise the retina for better vitreous shave. Second, it can be used indirectly to ascertain if the retina can be fully flatten, failure of which may suggest proliferative vitreoretinopathy (PVR), which then guide the surgeon with on the table surgical decision making. It can also serve as an indirect method to assess if the PVR membrane peel is adequate, as an inadequate membrane peel may still result in an unflattened retina under HL. Third, in rare cases, it can also be used as a temporising measure of retinal tamponade in complex VR cases requiring multiple VR surgery to complete the process.

11. In view of multiple breaks involving many quadrants, 360° very peripheral endolaser (with segmentation to prophylactically contain any imminent RD) is a sensible approach to reduce risk of a second operation for redetachment.

12. Then HL is aspirated through fluid–air exchange (FAX) at 40–60 mmHg initially (the higher the pressure, the faster it will drain). As the HL bubble gets smaller, the infusion pressure (of air) is reduced (to around 20 mmHg) to facilitate smoother HL bubble removal with the flute. The reason here is because as the bubble of HL gets smaller, the higher pressure will press on it and make the bubble flatter, and this will make removal of HL with the flute more challenging. The lesser pressure will result in a more spherical bubble of HL for easier removal with the flute. The usual pressure for air infusion is accepted at 20–30 mmHg, in preparation for air–gas exchange.

13. For this case, C3F8 14% gas was used for longer lasting tamponade. It is important to bear in mind the major gases used in VR surgery, including their vital characteristics. The table below will give some useful gas characteristics:

Characteristics	SF6	C2F6	C3F8
Expansion delay	1 day	1.5 days	3 days
Effective tamponade time	7 days	15 days	30 days
Presence of gas	15 days	30 days	60 days
Concentration of nonexpansile gas	20%	16%	12%
Rate of expansion	3	3.3	4

Table 1. Adapted from www.arcadophta.com/prod-gases_EN.html [9].

14. The intraocular pressure (IOP) should be checked as it is desirable to leave the high with a reasonable IOP (e.g., 20–25 mmHg).

15. The three-port sclerostomy sites are closed with 8 'O' vicryl sutures. The first two port sclerotomies are closed up with the 8 'O' vicryl suture first.

16. The third port (with the infusion line) is used to inject in the C3F8 14% gas. A 27G needle is used to release the air as C3F8 gas is being injected into the globe. It is important to continuously assess the IOP of the eye as the gas is being injected, to avoid an over-inflated eye.

17. Here, it is important to check the gas concentration and composition with the scrub nurse. Furthermore, as the retinal gas used is of a heavy molecule compared to air, it behaves like an 'invisible liquid', and as such, when connecting the gas containing syringe to the infusion cannula (through the three-way tap), it has to be done with the syringe orifice faced up. If the syringe orifice is tilted downwards as it is connected with the infusion cannula, this may result in some lost of the gas, making the gas diluted and rendering it less effective for the job it is intended to do in the globe.

18. Further gas top up intravitreally may be required after closing all three sclerostomy sites.

19. In our opinion, we prefer all three sclerostomy sites to be firmly secured with the sutures discussed above, to minimise any gas leak, which may make the surgical result less optimum.

20. Subconjunctival cefuroxime is our preferred choice of immediate post-operative antibiotics.

Further learning points:

1. Both C3F8 and silicone oil are shown to reduce rate of PVR.

2. It is important to note that retina must always be left flat after RD repair vitrectomy surgery in inferior break RD (as inferior detachment is a risk factor for redetachment and PVR), PVR, giant retinal tears (GRTs), and silicone oil cases.

3. Trocars nearer to 3 and 9 o'clock position will enable the surgeon to can get better access to 6 o'clock position especially in a big eye.

Case 2: Macula-on slowly progressing inferior RD with two small inferior retinal holes in the absence of PVD

This case was treated with indirect cryotherapy and sclera buckle.

1. Good clinical examination and drawing of the exact RD map utilising retinal vessel landmarks is necessary for a successful sclera buckle, which is preferably done under general anaesthesia (GA).

2. A 270° peritomy was performed, and the medial rectus (MR), lateral rectus (LR), and inferior rectus (IR) muscles were exposed and slung. The slinging of the recti muscles can be done by using 4 'O' silk. This is important for the manoeuvring of the globe in various positions to facilitate the indirect cryotherapy (cryo) and sclera buckling.

3. Although the RD may have been meticulously mapped out at the planning stage of the sclera buckle, it is always prudent to check for other breaks on the operating table, using the indirect ophthalmoscopy.

4. Indentation is then performed to see if the detached retina can be opposed on pressure for cryoreaction. If this is possible, then there is no need to drain the SRF using external approach. If this is not possible, then draining of the SRF may be considered. Cryo will inadvertently soften the eye.

5. It has been reported that retinal pigment epithelium (RPE) can still work in chronic detached retina.

6. A 5 'O' Ethibond-spatulated needle was used as anchor sutures for the buckle.

7. Buckle 277 is a broad buckle commonly used. It is 7 mm wide. Sutures are placed to anchor the buckle and are preplaced 9 mm wide allowing for tightening later and securing of the buckle.

8. It is important to check central retina artery (CRA) perfusion after the buckle has been secured. If the CRA is pulsating significantly, then paracentesis of the anterior chamber (AC) should be considered to lower the IOP.

Case 3: Superotemporal macula-off RD with superotemporal (S-T) breaks in the presence of PVD

1. This case was managed by three-port pars plana vitrecomy; the basic steps and considerations were discussed as above.

2. One of the aims of vitrectomy here is to release the tension of vitreous traction on the retina tear, especially the anterior lips of the retinal break. The approach to this is to do vitrectomy from the periphery moving slowly towards the anterior lips of the break, clearing the vitreous and thereby releasing the traction, from one end to the other end of the anterior lips of the break. The vitrector probe (once made inactive) can also be used to access if the break is cleared of all vitreous traction by touching on the borders of the break. If it is freely mobile without resistance, this suggests that there is no traction.

3. The vitrector can also be used to drain SRF through the retinal break as the vitrectomy surgery progresses.

4. After performing step 2, the retina may be flattened at this stage with HL.

5. HL (e.g., perfluorodecalin) can be used to fill up to the posterior aspect of the break to flatten and splint the retina for easier vitrectomy work near the retina and to achieve a thinner, more complete shave.

6. A 360° indentation is then performed to check for other breaks.

7. Then cryo of all the breaks are then done under saline (or under air which is the other option). Some surgeons prefer to use endodiathermy to highlight/mark the area of breaks for convenient identification for cryo.

8. FAX is then performed, with the backflush being held just above the break to drain the SRF so that the retina will flatten as the FAX is completed.

9. Removal of heavy liquid using the backflush or vitrector is then performed.

10. If there is a water tide/mark crease on the macula, this needs to be flattened or ironed out to avoid metamorphopsia. One option is to reintroduce heavy liquid from one side to the other to iron the retina flat, if this was discovered after FAX. The second option is for longer acting gas (e.g., C3F8 14%) and do face down posture for a day.

11. The pitfall here is to be able to distinguish pseudowater tide/mark crease from true crease. A water tide/mark could be actually the junction between oedematous detached retina, which had just been reattached and healthy retina (pseudocrease), and not a real crease as such. Therefore, this sign needs to be assessed carefully to decide if it is a true crease.

12. Gas injection and close up is standard procedure as described in Case 1.

Further learning points:

1. In cases where the RD is not bullous (i.e., shallow), HL may not be required, as macula folds is less likely, and any residual SRF can be absorbed by the RPE. Face down posture with gas-filled eye may be beneficial in such cases.

2. It can take 20 minutes for crystalline lens to get cloudy (depending on the degree of cataract present prior to surgery) with FAX air in vitreous cavity.

3. Longer acting gas means less PVR rate especially in Inferior RD cases.

Case 4: A 5-day history of inferior RD macula-off with a horse shoe tear of moderate size at 7 o'clock position with PVD present

1. This case required vitrectomy (basic steps and considerations as discussed previously).

2. In inferior RD, inferior vitreous needs to be very closely shaved to minimise tangential and sideway traction, which can lead to future redetachment and PVR.

3. With a horse shoe tear (anterior) flap, it is best to retinectomise the flap to make easier access of the break during SRF drainage by backflush. Furthermore, it may serve as a more effective and convenient way to relieve traction (since the flap can be considered as the anterior lip which is subjected to vitreous traction which caused the tear in the first place).

4. The break on this occasion is quite near the ora serrata. If backflush is blocked, then try to squeeze on the nozzle to try release any blockages. Reasons for a blocked backflush include thick vitreous catching on the probe (requiring further shaving) and the probe catching on the edge of the break when draining the SRF (requiring the probe to be placed higher and aim central to the break).

5. When draining SRF with backflush during FAX, the probe needs to be very steadily placed centrally in relation to the break as visualisation of the fundus is poor. If not observed, this may lead to an ineffective FAX, resulting in persistent SRF with the break still open.

6. Occasionally, it may not be possible to flatten retina due to extensive bullous RD. Then options include the following:

a. Use long-acting C3F8 14% gas with utilising the steam roller technique of posturing to milk out the SRF. An example is that if in the left eye, after RD repair, before closing up, there were still some SRF temporal to the macula, with a break temporal (2 o'clock position), the steam roller technique will require the patient to lie on the left cheek to pillow (so that the gas bubble will be exerting nasally) for half an hour, after which the patient will lie face down for another half hour (this will move the maximal exertion of the gas bubble from nasal to middle (macula) area of the retina. Then finally, the patient will lie with right cheek to pillow. This will result in the gas bubble having maximal exertion in the temporal region. In effect, this entire manoeuvre will slowly move the bubble maximal exertion point from nasal to middle to temporal, resulting in the milking effect of the SRF to expel through the temporal side opening). This effect is akin to a steam roller concept and hence the name of this manoeuvre.

b. Use HL (under air or saline) and redrain the SRF before introducing C3F8 14% gas.

c. Make a retinotomy at the most superior point (highest point) accessible for draining the SRF and then cryo to the retinotomy site.

These options are not exhaustive and merely highlight the versatility of VR surgery, whereby decision making on the table is crucial, and is dictated on a case by case basis.

Further learning points:

1. After 1 week of inferior RD usually PVR will start.

2. The prognosis of macula-off RD of less than 1 week will have a better prognosis than after 1 week RD.

3. In general, studies had shown that the major risk factors for increased risk of retinal redetachment include inferior break RD and PVR. Therefore, the decision on the appropriate approach to manage inferior RD needs to take into consideration multiple factors, as the surgeon and patient will have to live with the decision made. The factors taken into consideration will depend on the visual potential, macula-on or macula-off RD, presence or absence of PVR, and position of RD. If, for example, the case is an inferior RD with break at 6 o'clock position, with macula-off and PVR that could not be flatten with HL despite removal of some PVR membranes, then we can consider retinectomy, peripheral endolaser, and silicone oil and cryo at each end of the retinectomy site. For the retinectomy to work, this should be performed for 180° with retinectomy relieving incisions at each end. The relieving incisions at each end will reduce the risk of further PVR progression as it limits the expansion of PVR membranes. If there is more visual potential with macula-on inferior RD, then we will consider cryo, gas, and buckle. The buckle here will serve as an enhanced indentation site against which the retinal break can be firmly opposed while allowing for the cryoreaction to take place in 5–7 days. In fresh inferior breaks, buckle may not be necessary. The reason to avoid silicone oil in an inferior RD with good visual potential is that it can actually cause issues like IOP and macula toxicity leading to reduced vision.

4. If there are multiple inferior breaks RD, depending on severity, there are several management options, although the list below is not exhaustive and aim at stimulating the decision-making process of the new VR surgeons.

5. Possible options depending on severity are as follows (increasing severity of inferior RD):

a. Vitrectomy, cryo gas

b. Vitrectomy, cryo, gas, buckle (e.g., 277 buckle), e.g., two breaks and difficulty trimming the vitreous gel at the edge of the breaks.

c. Vitrectomy, cryo, oil—e.g., PVR grades B/C

d. Vitrectomy, cryo, oil, and buckle—e.g., macula reasonable prognosis

e. Vitrectomy, cryo/retinectomy and oil—e.g., PVR grades B/C with peeling of star membrane. This is appropriate for cases of poor prognosis of visual acuity less than 6/36 Snellen.

Note: SRF drainage through an accessible break can be with or without heavy liquid, in saline or in air.

Case 5: A patient with PVD positive and an almost total RD with inferior breaks ×2

No PVR was found.

After the basic vitrectomy, the technique used here is by filling HL up to the two inferior breaks (which is very periphery) to fill the entire vitreous cavity, thus pushing most of the SRF away. Now the retina will be flat, and the breaks can then be treated with cryo or laser retinopexy. Then FAX is switched on. This means that at this point, the vitreous cavity has three interface systems, namely, air, fluid, and HL. During the FAX, the backflush or aspirating vitrector is placed at the fluid level (which is in between the air and the HL layer), to drain all the fluid making it a two interface system (Air and HL). Then the infusion cannula is removed from the trocar to drain out infusion fluid and HL, which may be contained in the infusion line through the FAX mode. If this step is not done, there is a theoretical risk that some fluid and HL may be present, and continuing with the FAX may result in some fluid and/or HL being reinserted into the vitreous cavity. This in turn may get through the retinal break causing an SRF accumulation, which is not ideal. Then the infusion cannula is reinserted into the trocar. Next, with FAX mode, HL–air exchange is done. As there is no fluid on top of the heavy liquid, it was not mandatory to put backflush near the break to drain. After FAX, air–gas exchange is performed, prior to closing up.

Case 6: A young man with traumatic macula hole and chronic macula-off almost total RD

It is postulated that PVR was not present despite chronicity due to non-PVD and the firm vitreous is keeping pigments away.

After the standard vitrectomy, the following steps were taken:

1. Inducing PVD in a young patient can be challenging. One method is to activate continuous suction with circular motion outwardly for two rounds before lifting up the vitreous body. The light pipe can be used to shine on the shadow of the vitreous body to confirm PVD induction. This method can be repeated until PVD obtained. Membrane blue and triamcinolone can be used to highlight vitreous body. Central PVD in this case does not necessarily mean peripheral PVD in the young, which need to be carefully induced, to avoid retina capture on vitrector orifice, which should be pointed 180° away from the retina surface.

2. Internal limiting membrane (ILM) in traumatic cases and in the young can be VERY challenging as it is very sticky and difficult to peel. For macula work, the surgeon must ensure appropriate readjustment of depth perception for the higher magnified macula lens, to avoid retinal touch.

To peel in this case, the force of the forceps should be concentrated sideways along the surface of the retina before lifting up to ensure a significant amount of membrane can be peeled off at any one time, which can be another challenge in view of the mobile retina.

3. If macula hole is too small, consider superior accessible retinotomy site (above the equator) for drainage of SRF.

4. Since this case had no PVR, and the retina can be flattened, long-acting gas (C3F8 14% is used prior to closing up.

Case 7: Inferior RD with early PVR, and with a history of previous RD repair surgery and removal of silicone oil procedure

1. In this case, the approach is inferior retinectomy 180° with relaxing retinectomy. The role of radial relaxing retinectomy (which can be made in several locations as the condition dictates) is to help flatten PVR retina and reduce risk of future PVR formation.

2. After retinectomy, heavy liquid can be used to flatten retina before application of peripheral laser retinopexy. Then FAX followed by silicone oil insertion. When silicone oil is filled, there may be some residual fluid trapped between the silicone oil and the iris lens diaphragm. This can be aspirated with backflush after removal of the infusion line, which may contain more fluid/heavy liquid. If the infusion line is not removed prior to aspiration of residual fluid, this may result in reintroduction of residual fluid into the vitreous cavity when the infusion line is finally removed.

Further learning points:

1. Retinectomy can cause haemorrhage if retinal or choroid vessels are involved. As the choroid is the most vascularised tissue in the body, the haemorrhage with the involvement of choroidal vessels can be very significant.

2. When performing retinectomy with the vitrector, it is prudent to ensure that the cutter is held just on the layer of the retina being retinectomised as any deeper will invariably shear the choroidal vessels leading to significant haemorrhage. Bottle height can go up to 80 mmHg to tamponade the haemorrhage, if this was to happen.

3. A small strand of retina connecting the anterior and posterior aspect of the retinectomy site left behind in retinectomy for PVR can cause further PVR and retinal detachment. As such, there is a need to make sure that all retina in the path of retinectomy be completely removed.

Case 8: Proliferative diabetic retinopathy (PDR) with vitreous haemorrhage with previous pan-retinal photocoagulation (PRP)

1. PVD induction in such cases can be very challenging. The following approach can be used based on the level of difficulty in inducing PVD (in ascending order of difficulty) as follows:

-Persistent and repeated circular motion in aspiration using the vitrector (with cutter mode off) around the vitreous body near to the optic disc is performed. Always aim the vitrector away from the macula and work around the disc. Disc area-induced PVD is considered complete PVD. For this reason, the need to ascertain anatomy of macula and disc is of paramount importance and can be challenging with suboptimal view in vitreous haemorrhage cases. Working away from macula sweeping around the disc with the vitrector, pulling towards the midperipheral retina before lifting the hyaloid face, is one suggested approach. It has to be noted that these steps need to be repeated until a full PVD is achieved, failure of which may result in further fibrosis with possible tractional RD (TRD) and recurrent vitreous haemorrhage.

-The vitrector aspiration rate can be increased further in more adherent hyaloids face cases.

-In cases where hyaloids face is not readily visible, membrane blue can be considered, as this will stain the hyaloids face enough for visualisation, to ensure complete separation from the retina both centrally and in the midperiphery.

-The use of triamcinolone is another alternative to membrane blue for visualisation of the hyaloids face.

-Physical manual separation of posterior vitreous face with MVR (micro vitreoretinal) blade, ILM forceps, scissors (20G) which can be right angle or curved.

The listed approaches above can be used repeatedly and in combination in very difficult cases until PVD is achieved.

If vitreous gel is left behind in the posterior pole/macula region, then rhegmatogenous RD and/ or TRD will eventually ensue.

2. Organised haemorrhage near the retina can technically be removed using backflush, again pulling away from the macula. If one end of the organised haemorrhage is not budging, then the surgeon can try removing the complex from another end.

3. Haemorrhage can be tamponade by increasing bottle height or increasing infusion pressure. If source of bleeding can be found, the surgeon can consider endocautery.

4. Macula lens can be used to increase magnification for close work around the macula or in difficult to induced PVD.

Further points to consider:

1. Do not pull to induce PVD at the retinal blood vessels arcades.

2. If peripheral shave is done but PVD is not yet induced at the posterior pole, this will lead to rhegmatogenous RD if left alone. If PVD is induced at this stage (after peripheral vitreous shave is done), it will spring up to the ora serrata, and the whole process of peripheral shave needs to be started again. Therefore, it is crucial to induce PVD in such cases at the posterior pole for a subsequent complete core and peripheral vitrectomy in a time efficient manner.

3. Ala-Sil (Altomed) can be used in place of balanced salt solution (BSS) in vitrectomy/ delamination cases, which have significant active vitreous haemorrhage, as this infusion

material will not mix with blood and let the blood stay in a loculated place as the surgeon continues with vitrectomy work without making the view hazy from the haemorrhage.

4. Bucket-handle technique: In cases where parts of the posterior pole are affected by TRD, core vitrectomy should be followed by relieving traction at the TRD site (with delamination as required) and then followed by the PVD induction in the posterior pole. If core vitrectomy and peripheral vitrectomy shave are performed without posterior pole PVD, this may result in fibrovascular TRD flattening, as the anteroposterior tractional force had been relieved from the core and peripheral shave vitrectomy. This will lead to insufficient vitreous body left for engaging with the vitrector to continue with the process of vitrectomy/delamination work. Furthermore, it will be more difficult to perform delamination of the fibrovascular attachments in a flattened TRD complex. This principle is known as the bucket-handle technique as the 'handle' represents the fibrovascular traction bands.

Case 9: Temporal GRT with PVD positive and macula-off

Learning points:

-GRT is defined at a peripheral retinal break of 3 or more clock hours.

-Such cases require good peripheral shave and relieving traction, just as any case of rhegmatogenous RD.

-HL is used to flatten the retina, followed by endolaser of the GRT. For places hard to reach at either end of the GRT, cryo can be used to join the endolaser to the ora serrata.

-GRT is a recognised risk of the development of PVR, and hence silicone oil should be considered, even in macula-on cases.

For this particular case, when FAX was done to remove heavy liquid, the retina ballooned out, and retina slippage occurred. In this case, FAX was stopped, and heavy liquid was reintroduced. This flattened the retina. Backflush was used to aspirate the remaining SRF, the position of the backflush being as near to the posterior lip (near where the endolaser marks were). This action can also facilitate the retina to reposition from the slippage position to its original position but should not be done forcefully.

Variation of techniques to inject silicone oil: One option is for heavy liquid–air–oil exchange (with hand 1 holding the light pipe and hand 2 holding the backflush). This technique can pose a higher risk of retinal slippage. Another option is using chandelier light in the fourth (30G) port, with hand 1 holding the backflush and hand 2 holding the silicon oil infusion cannula and the three-way tap on the main infusion line connected to one of the three trocars is switched off at the same time.

One method of minimising catching on the retinal edge of break while aspirating using backflush is to close the aspirating hole of the backflush until it is aligned out of the way of the retina break edges, before reopening to aspirate further.

Therefore, it is important to pay close attention to the retina position in such cases to observe for any retina slippage during FAX. With experience, one can tell the difference between oedematous retina and crinkling of retina.

Furthermore, in such cases, it is prudent to consider a direct silicone oil–heavy liquid direct exchange. Since the normal infusion tube (which connects from the three-way tap to the trocar) is not strong enough to withstand the pressure from the silicone oil injector (which can be as high as 30lbs/sq inch, equivalent to 1500 mmHg), a special silicone oil tubing is used to substitute the original infusion tube. This will allow for both hands of the surgeon to work on the retina.

NB: Decision making during surgery is crucial and one has to think of few steps ahead.

Case 10: Total RD with PVD positive in a phakic patient

In this case, it was a chronic RD. However, only two small peripheral holes were seen, one at 1 o'clock and another at 8 o'clock. The detached retina was still mobile. Since the holes were small, it was postulated that the pigment cells would be difficult to make their way to the vitreous cavity, which explained why there were no PVR.

-In the presence of PVD, when doing vitrectomy, in view of the mobile retina, we can consider HL to splint the retina for a more stable vitrectomy shave.

-Small holes are difficult to visualise, so such breaks are preferably cryoed in saline. The other alternative is to endocautery mark the breaks and cryo under air.

-In phakic eyes, decision sometimes need to be made, when the lens get cloudy. In this case, options are (1) to perform cataract surgery and lens implant and continue with the retinal work with a better fundal view and (2) consider after cryo/laser to the area/s of break/s, to fill in with silicone oil. The rationale behind this is that under silicone oil, small breaks that may have been missed may remain stable. If the cataract developed further over the course of several months, then the surgeon can perform combined cataract extraction and lens implant (phaco+IOL) and removal of silicone oil (ROSO) and at that stage reexamine the retina and treat any breaks found.

Case 11: Right macula-off temporal bullous RD with multiple small peripheral breaks

In bullous RD cases, the aim is as follows:

-Core and peripheral vitrectomy

-Vitrectomising near the major breaks (while being cautious about vacuum (low) and cut rate (high)) in order to remove any traction and allowing SRF to come through in order to flatten the retina thereby stabilising and controlling the retinal position. Care must be taken to avoid iatrogenic retinal breaks.

-PVD is then induced (if PVD not present).

-The surgeon will aim to achieve as thin a peripheral shave as possible.

-While doing vitrectomy in such cases, one can expect bullous retina coming and going depending on the position of the eye and vitrector. This is due to the dynamic fluid movement depending on the position of the vitrector. One can consider using HL to stabilise the retina in such cases.

-The small breaks can be cryoed (or lasered) under saline or air (surgeon dependent)

-Then FAX is started, with drainage through the main small break being performed using the vitrector initially and revert to backflush, for a more refined and controlled aspiration of the residual fluid in the vitreous cavity. Once the fluid level during the FAX dropped below the retina break being drained, the backflush can then be moved to the area just above the optic disc to complete the FAX.

-If one should refill the vitreous cavity with BSS after FAX especially in the myopic eye (for any technical reasons, e.g., retinal folds near macula), one must be aware not to put too much vacuum on the vitrector initially, as there will be a lag of air in the infusion line before BSS comes through, creating vacuum to cause 'kissing retina'. During the beginning of this process, instruments need to be held high up in the vitreous cavity, as the sudden 'kissing retina' effect may damage the retina, on sudden forceful contact with the instruments if those were at the base of the posterior pole.

-Should FAX result in reformation of bullous retina, then this may suggest that fluid has reentered the break, possibly from suboptimal drainage technique, or original break is too small to effectively drain through or a loculated SRF collection, and the options for further procedure are as follows:

a. Refill vitreous cavity with BSS and perform an accessible retinotomy, and perform FAX and drained through the new retinotomy site. Then contiguous cryo on the multiple small breaks under air performed (may consider diathermy to mark, or draw map of breaks) (applicable to loculated SRF collection and/or treated small breaks, pertaining to this case).

b. HL to flatten retina and 360° laser retinopexy. (This can be an option in situation with RD but no breaks found.)

Further learning points to consider:

There are many cryotherapy machines for VR work. Occasionally, the cryo probe is not responsive. Therefore, the surgeon needs to be aware of basic troubleshooting. This includes the following: (a) check to see if the probe itself is working by testing first, (b) check for leaking probe, and (c) check to see if the cylinder is empty.

Case 12: Inferior break developing during ROSO requiring cryo and refill with silicone oil

The decision on how to proceed in such case depends upon the presence or absence of PVR and the assessment of individual patient's circumstances, e.g., requiring more ops, etc. Possible options include the following:

-Cryo and/or laser and long-acting gas with positioning in the absence of PVR.

-Cryo and/or laser and refill with silicone oil if no PVR.

-Laser and retinectomy with silicone oil if PVR.

-May require PVR membrane removal.

Case 13: Inferior macula-off RD with previous RD repair vitrectomy surgery over 5 years ago

Learning points:

-Retinal break can still be adjacent to the cryoed area.

-Main reason of RD in this case is due to inadequate vitreous shave during the first RD repair. Thick base of vitreous left behind from the initial surgery can still have the potential to undergo peripheral PVD leading to new retinal breaks.

-Redo in this case involved a much thinner shave especially at the area of break.

-In this case, the break was impossible to find on cursory indentation. The subretinal ILM blue chimney smoke method was used after heavy liquid insertion, to avoid ILM blue to go under the macula. The ILM blue dye was injected with a 40G needle in the subretinal layer of the RD. Then gentle indentation and milking to look for the leaking dye, which shall be the area of small break where it leaked dye. Subretinal dye should ideally drained out once it served its purpose, and in this case, retinotomy was done before draining out the dye, since 40G hole is too small to effectively drain the dye, after the identification and treatment of the break.

-Since there were no PVR, long-acting gas and posturing face down for 3 days was the decision made in this case.

-With PVR, the surgeon may be required to perform a 180° retinectomy and relieving retinotomy and enolaser and silicone oil.

Case 14: Inferior RD with macula involvement, but multiple holes in all quadrants in a 38-year-old man

-PVD induction can be tricky in the younger patients who had not naturally developed PVD. In detached retina, PVD induction is done by pulling vitreous body towards area of detachment to the periphery before pulling up. If PVD induction is only concentrated on the centre, this will only achieve partial PVD and, hence, the motion of going from central to peripheral before pulling up the vitreous body to induce a complete PVD.

-Multiple breaks will require 360° laser retinopexy. Since no PVR in this case, long-acting gas was used (instead of silicone oil).

-During FAX to remove heavy liquid and fluid, the surgeon must also go near the break to drain SRF as well, to aim to achieve a flat retina. In this case, there was a sequestered SRF pocket near the macula. Retinotomy was done to drain the SRF to achieve a flat retina. The retinotomy site in this case was not near the periphery, and hence laser retinopexy (and not cryo—since the cryo probe could not reach the retinotomy site due to its location) was used.

Case 15: Redo inferior retinal detachment in a 40-year-old man

In this case, the issue was that of an inadequately treated (cryo) break. This break was cryoed, and since there was no PVR, long-acting gas was put in place. The learning point here is to ensure that adequate cryo is applied to the break in the primary surgery through meticulous observation.

Case 16: Redo inferior RD in a 70-year-old lady

In this case, there were signs of PVR grade B. There were no collagenous membranes to peel.

Even in Grade B PVR, there can be radial shortening of the retina, in that after retinectomy was done, the shortening can be very significant. In this case, the retina contracted centrally with its new retinectomised border settled near to the major retinal vessel arcades.

In this case, silicone oil was used, after air/heavy liquid exchange. The silicone oil was injected separately from hand 2 with hand 1 holding the light pipe (this procedure was previously discussed above).

Case 17: Diabetic retinopathy fibrovascular traction requiring delamination

Bucket-handle technique utilised here. This means no full vitrectomy in this case, with only enough vitrectomy to get at the posterior hyaloid face (PHF), as full vitrectomy will release traction and hence flatten the traction area, making it difficult to release and remove more membranes.

The approach to delamination can be performed by using the 20G curve scissors (although a curved 23G scissors can also be used) and go underneath the PHF and with the scissors opened, lift up the PHF and cut, so as to minimise the chances of cutting the retina creating a tear. This will create a surgical plane for lifting the membrane complex en bloc. When the scissors are closed, they can be used as a pick to tease up the PHF.

Sometimes despite the best efforts, retina break/hole cannot be avoided. Usually, this happens in the areas just near the arcades and sometimes near the temporal macula region. This is best treated with laser retinopexy. The closer it is to the macula, the lighter the laser should be applied. In the unlikely anatomy position of papillomacular bundle tear/break, this is best left alone. In any case, expansile gas is used and face down posture adopted for 1–2 days.

The objective in TRD is to relieve the traction at the strongest adhesion point/s via delamination. Thereafter, once complete PVD is induced, then we can continue straight to complete the vitrectomy.

Pirouetting and moving the fundal view in opposite directions of vector of rotating the eye will increase periphery view. Cutting as close to the edge of view is recommended for a thin vitreous shave. In areas of vitreous base haemorrhage which cannot be removed, in the area of entry site, one can consider external cryo behind the site to reduce risk of entry site break.

Case 18: Superonasal bullous macula-off retinal detachment with PVD positive

Heavy liquid is key is the splinting of such cases.

Extra macula fold can still occur after FAX if the heavy liquid is not filled up to the level of just below the posterior border of the retinal break.

Technically, as long as the three interface (air, fluid, and HL) can be changed to two interface (air and HL), and no fluid getting into the break, then we should be able to avoid retinal slip and /or retinal folds (which is caused by residual fluid in the vitreous cavity.

Retinal folds post operatively usually does not cause much visual symptoms to patients unless it is a macula fold. To reoperate, one can use a 40G needle to inject BSS subretinal to create a bullous RD to extend into the macula area where the fold is. Then use HL to flatten out the retina, ironing out the macula fold at the same time. Retinotomy may be required in the periphery to drain out the SRF and finishing off with gas fill and to close up.

Case 19: Inferior retinal detachment with an inferior moderate size break, who opted to wait over the weekend prior to surgery, resulting in early membrane PVR, but macula-on

This case is rare as usually PVR cases are associated with macula-off (which means different approach to management).

Learning points:

It has been documented that certain genetics, e.g., HLA DR4 can be associated with propensity for PVR development.

In this case, even a wait of 4–5 days (as opposed to 2 days) can already result in PVR membrane formation.

In such cases while operating, one must actively look out for early PVR and assess mobility of the detached retina. Early PVR can be stiff, although it may retain limited mobility. The other feature to look out for is retinal folds that will not change shape within a relatively mobile retinal detachment. The approach to such case is to use an MVR blade (25G to enter 23G trocar) splice the membrane to unfold the retina. Another method of assessing stiffness in equivocal case is to use HL to see if this can completely flatten the retina.

The management decision for this case is as follows:

a. Inferior PVR macula-on: try to release adhesions of retinal folds by splicing PVR membranes to unfold retina. If SRF drainage can flatten the detached retina, long-acting gas and face down posture can be utilised. If retina is not properly flattened, a buckle can be added to increase success (added indentation to counter the shortened retina).

b. If this case redetached, we may then consider laser retinopexy and buckle, after getting rid of more membranes. Silicone oil should not be used in primary RD repair case in this situation due to macula toxicity (as the case is macula-on). The buckle acts to shorten the anterior vitreous base to reduce traction, and also act as a good addition to tamponade.

c. If after the above approach (a and b) but the retina redetached, we may then consider retinectomy and silicone oil (last resort).

d. However, if the macula was off (pertaining to this case), we may consider silicone oil in the first instance.

The above approaches are dependent on the state of the eye as discussed above. It serves as a prelude to the reader to utilise lateral thinking in the decision making in VR surgery.

Case 20: Inferior retinal detachment with two inferior breaks at 6 o'clock and PVR grade B, in a background of pseudoxanthoma elasticum (PXE), who had cataract surgery about 3 months ago

This was treated with vitrectomy, cryo, 360° laser retinopexy, and inferior buckle.

-PXE can be a predisposing factor for retinal breaks due to weaker connective tissue. In this case, there were a few superior breaks but without RD.

-It is important to recognise the PVR at an early stage, which can manifest as crinkling of the retina (blood vessels crinkling can be a good clue of early PVR). PVR can be anterior or posterior or both. In the prevalence of PVR types, posterior is more common than anterior. Anterior PVR traction forces are A-P, circumferential and anterior perpendicular traction, where posterior PVR can take more random vectors. The objective in nonsheath PVR is to release any traction and to flatten as much the retina as possible, by cutting adhesions using MVR blade. Heavy liquid can be used to stabilise the retina and at the same time test the retina to see if it flattens —if not flattened, this suggests PVR adhesions still strong and require further adhesion relief.

The European VR Society RD Study (report 2) suggested that in cases of PVR requiring vitrectomy, a supplemental buckle may not be useful. http://www.aaojournal.org/article/S0161-6420(13)00102-4/pdf

http://www.eyecalcs.com/DWAN/pages/v6/v6c058.html

-In this case, inferior buckle is also used. This serves two purposes, one being to reduce the circumference and area of the PVR region in the hope of stabilising the flattened retina in that area. The second reason is to give additional tamponade to ensure closure of the breaks is permanent. While doing buckling, the IOP should not be high. One can consider filling the eye with heavy liquid to a high point in the eye to ensure globe maintenance during buckling. This means the infusion cannula can be temporarily disengaged, to make enough room for the buckling. Once buckling is done (using 277 broad band buckle), 360° laser retinopexy (in view of multiple breaks in all quadrants) and cryo are utilised.

-NB: Cryo machine should be set up prior to it being required. This is to ensure that cryo is not only set up once it is needed, as the warming up of machine and self-calibration takes time, and can mean that when one uses the probe to indent with the view to cryo breaks found, the cryo can go 'on' as part of the calibration process, thereby throwing the probe into uncontrolled freezing in undesired area. In this case, one option is to disconnect the probe from the machine or to cut with scissors the infusion line of the probe.

Case 21: A 67-year-old man with epiretinal membrane (ERM)

He is pseudophakic with anterior capsular phimosis.

In this case, ERM peel using diamond duster scrapper could not induce a flap, as this ERM happened to be a double membrane and firmly attached (like chewing gum) whereby the diamond dusted scrapper will only make the tissue bunched up without inducing a flap. In this case, using an MVR blade to scrape away from the surgeon (so as to have a view of tissue control at all times) to induce a flap. Sometimes, inevitably partial thickness retina layer maybe peeled of as the flap is induced. This should not cause much visual symptoms postoperative anecdotally. If the flap is friable and not able to be extended, then attempt to create another flap adjacent to it, so that the second flap can join the first flap to create a bigger flap before peeling. In this case, restaining with dual blue multiple times for better visualisation is helpful. Staining and restaining especially in double ERM layers will make each layer more discernable.

Usually, after initial staining, always look out for natural creases of the ERM which maybe prominent on primary staining. These creases can be used to create flaps and start the peel. It is better to peel off the ILM as well, if possible, to reduce the risk of ERM recurring (as ILM is the scaffold upon which the ERM proliferates).

The ERM membrane pegging to the retinal surface can be unpredictably anywhere (not neatly arranged) and peeling ERM will depend on the feel of least resistance. ILM peel on behaves more like an anterior capsulorrhexis during cataract phacoemulsification.

Case 22: A GRT repaired with cryo and 360° laser retinopexy and silicone-filled eye over 7 months, who had an ROSO, and during the procedure, inferior RD was noted

In this case, it should be treated like an RD. The inferior RD SRF was extensive, with the break appeared to be on the previous laser retinopexy site. FAX used to drain the SRF ended up with an inferior collection of SRF (with closure of the break). Hence, a retinotomy was performed under air. Retinotomy under air is more challenging, requiring aspiration to engage the retina before cutting to make the retinotomy. By using a backflush, SRF drainage was attempted but only able to achieve partial drainage. At this point, silicone oil was refilled. Despite silicone oil refilled, the SRF was still present. At this point, the idea was to use heavy liquid under the oil. A small proportion of oil was removed using the backflush, with the infusion line attached to one of the trocars. The HL was injected under the oil which flattened the retina. Then laser retinopexy was performed. The next step will be to remove the HL as top up silicone oil was injected. An independent silicon oil cannula was connected directly into the trocar, replacing the original infusion cannula, so that the surgeon is able to use the foot pedal to control the oil injection, while one hand holding the light pipe and the other holding the backflush to drain the HL. This is one unusual scenario when direct oil-HL exchange was performed.

Case 23: A total RD with Grade B PVR, with the nasal and superior part of RD not able to be flattened by HL

The approach in this case is as follows:

-Wide angle viewing system

-High-speed cutter

-Encirclage (for grade C PVR and above) to shortened the retina

-PFCL heavy liquid to try flatten the retina

-Membrane peel

-Retinectomy and laser/cryo (please note that this is best done with inferior 180°), and it is unusual to do retinectomy as a primary RD procedure

-Tamponade

NB: In cases of PVR where close vitreous shave is required, one can consider the 'proportional reflux dissection' on a 25+ G cutter. This cutter can be a multifunction effect depending on the adjustment of certain parameters. With this, the sphere of influence is smaller and less likely to cause iatrogenic break, in PVR membrane peeling.

In this case, after membrane peel, a nasal retinectomy in an attempt to flatten the retina was attempted. However, there is extensive haemorrhage despite diathermy before retinectomy. In view of the poor view, surgery stopped and eye filled up to max, to revisit (as a two-stage procedure) in 24–48 hours (any longer will cause IOP increased and inflammation ++). This approach flattened the retina and settled the haemorrhage, for the surgery to be completed.

Case 24: Vitreomacular traction (VMT) with visual distortion

Vitreous can be very sticky in such cases, and even though there is a Weiss ring, vitreous can still be firmly attached to macula. The approach in inducing PVD in this situation is to pull vitreous around the macula and never work on the fovea directly.

Membrane blue or triamcinolone can be used to confirm that vitreous is removed.

Paediatrics VR consideration:

-In paediatrics VR cases, the vitrectomy is just core vitrectomy as inducing a PVD would be disastrous to the very young retina.

Even in cases of retinopathy of prematurity (ROP), releasing traction is the main aim and not to remove majority of the vitreous.

The trocar approach to paediatric VR up to 15 years old is 2.5–3 mm behind limbus.

Case 25: Previous inferior retinectomy and silicone oil and ROSO presented with a redetachment

Inferotemporal area of retinectomy is found to have PVR lifting that area creating a break for RD to develop (macula-off almost total RD).

-Heavy liquid (HL) sequestered superiorly SRF, which means no breaks in the sequestered area.

Recognising straight (and unusual retinal detachment patterns) is important. This is caused by PVR. The source of traction/pulling effect needed to be worked out and then released, so that it will resume normal break contour, after which, laser retinopexy can be considered (either under HL or oil). In this case, it was decided to do under oil. The localised haemorrhage happened as a result of removing the fibrous adhesions.

Case 26: RD repaired (temporal) with silicone oil

ROSO was then performed and 5 months later developed this patient developed macula-off RD and PVD.

Learning points:

Retinectomy joining temporal breaks can be done in the superior peripheral arches 180°.

Case 27: Diabetic TRD

If sheets of hyaloid in posterior pole are left behind, this will invariably worsen the TRD leading to blindness and phthisical eye. Therefore, it is imperative to remove all the hyaloids sheets especially within the arcade of the macula. If outside the macula arcade, small islands can be left behind if too adherent to remove, as small islands do not have the tendency to contract to cause TRD (as it is not connected or networked with other islands of posterior pole hyaloids).

When delaminating, there is a need to quickly establish a surgical plane separating hyaloids from the fibrovascular tissue. Iatrogenic breaks can be laser pexied and drained to flat if possible (under heavy liquid)—in such cases, silicone oil needs to be considered. There may be a need to try different direction of peel for a good hyaloids peel.

4. Conclusion

This chapter describes the basic skills and pitfalls to avoid in VR surgery, which we hope will be especially useful to the novice and intermediate-level VR surgeons. The advanced VR surgeons may also find this chapter useful with some innovative surgical approach.

The above cases would have represented most of the VR case mix that the average VR surgeon will encounter in their daily practice. We hope that after reading this chapter, this will serve as a platform for further reading and practice, to improve the standards of VR surgery and enhancing patient safety and surgical outcomes of the readers.

Author details

Lik Thai Lim* and Ahmed El-Amir

*Address all correspondence to: likthai@gmail.com

Dear Authors, please add affiliations, Country

References

[1] Eckardt C. Transconjunctival sutureless 23-gauge vitrectomy. Retina 2005;25:208-11.

[2] Fujii GY, De Juan E Jr., Humayun MS, et al. A new 25-gauge instrument system for transconjunctival sutureless vitrectomy surgery. Ophthalmology 2002; 109:1807-12.

[3] Ibarra MS, Hermel M, Prenner JL, Hassan TS. Longer-term outcomes of transconjunctival sutureless 25-gauge vitrectomy. Am J Ophthalmol 2005;139:831-6.

[4] Lakhanpal RR, Humayun MS, De Juan E Jr., et al. Outcomes of 140 consecutive cases of 25-gauge transconjunctival surgery for posterior segment disease. Ophthalmology 2005;112:817-24.

[5] Oshima Y, Wakabayashi T, Sato T, Ohji M, Tano Y. A 27-gauge instrument system for transconjunctival sutureless microincision vitrectomy surgery. Ophthalmology. 2010;117:93-102.

[6] Oshima Y, Wakabayashi T, Sato T, et al. 13. Oshima Y, Wakabayashi T, Sato T, et al. A 27-gauge instrument system for transconjunctival sutureless microincision vitrectomy surgery. Ophthalmology. 2010;117:93-102.

[7] Sakaguchi H, Oshima Y, Nishida K, Awh CC. A 29/30-gauge dual-chandelier illumination system for panoramic viewing during microincision vitrectomy surgery. Retina. 2011;31:1231-1233Ophthalmology. 2010;117:93-102.

[8] Sakaguchi H, Oshima Y, Nishida K, Awh CC. A 29/30-gauge dual-chandelier illumination system for panoramic viewing during microincision vitrectomy surgery. Retina. 2011;31:1231-1233

[9] www.arcadophta.com/prod-gases

7

Trabeculotomy Augmented by Postoperative Topical Medications vs. Trabeculectomy Augmented by Mitomycin C

Hiroshi Kobayashi

Abstract

Purpose: To study the safety and hypotensive effect of trabeculotomy augmented by postoperative topical medical treatment in patients with open-angle glaucoma and to compare with trabeculectomy augmented by mitomycin C.

Methods: Inanon-randomized consecutive case series, we studied 82 patients with open-angle glaucoma who underwent trabeculotomyaugmented by postoperative medical therapy or trabeculectomy augmented with Mitomycin C. Forty-two patients underwent trabeculotomyfollowed by latanoprost 0.004%, timololmaleate XE 0.5% and brinzolamide 1% and 40 patients underwent trabeculectomy augmented with Mitomycin C. Patients were followed-up for 12 months and a success rate based on intraocular pressure was compared.

Results: Mean baseline intraocular pressure was27.9 ± 5.4 mmHg in the trabeculotomy group and 28.3 ± 4.2 mmHg in the trabeculectomy group (P = 0.7). Mean postoperative intraocular pressure was 15.1 ± 2.1 mmHg at 3 months, 14.7 ± 2.1 mmHg at 6 months, and 14.9 ± 2.0 mmHg at 12 months in the trabeculotomy group and 12.2 ± 1.9 mmHg at 3 months, 12.8 ± 3.0 mmHg at 6 months, and 13.9 ± 4.2mmHg at 12 months in the trabeculectomy group.Mean intraocular pressure in the trabeculotomygroup was significantly higher than that in the trabeculectomy group at 3 and 6 months (P < 0.0001 at 3 months; P = 0.0005 at 6 months) and there was no significant difference between the two groups at 12 months (P = 0.1). At 12 months, 42 patients (100%) in the trrabeculotomy group and 37 patients (92.5 %) in the traberculectomy group achieved an intraocular pressure of less than or equal to 20 mmHg and a minimum of 30 percent reduction (P = 0.1). In the trabeculectomy group, 15 patients

(37.5 %) received laser suture lysis,6 patients (15.0 %) underwent needling procedure, and 3 patients (7.5 %) underwent additional surgery, although no patient in the trabeculotomy group received postoperative intervention except for topical medical treatment. In the trabeculotomy group, patients with higher preoperative intraocular pressure showed a significantly higher intraocular pressure at 12 months postoperatively ($P < 0.0001$), although there was no significant correlation between them in the trabeculectomy group.

Conclusions: There was no significant difference in hypotensive efficacy between patients undergoing trabeculotomyaugmented by postoperative topical medications and those undergoing trabeculectomyaugmented by Mitomycin Cat 12 months. In those receiving trabeculotomy, patients with higher preoperative intraocular pressure showed a significantly higher intraocular pressure at 12 months even though less than 20 mmHg.

Keywords: trabeculotomy, trabeculectomy, postoperative medication

1. Introduction

Trabeculectomy has been a standard procedure for medically uncontrollable glaucoma [1]. Serious postoperative complications are not infrequently associated with trabeculectomy [2-5]. These include flat anterior chamber, hypotony and choroidal detachment caused by overfiltration, late-onset bleb-related complications, including endophthalmitis, and cataract progression. Shigeeda et al. demonstrated that 44.5% of patients who had undergone trabeculectomy augmented with mitomycin C showed a success defined as an intraocular pressure of less than 16 mm Hg after 8 years [6]. However, Tanihara et al. demonstrated that medical treatment following trabeculotomy provided an additional intraocular pressure reduction and that this surgery produced long-term stability of intraocular pressure control [7]. Trabeculotomy infrequently causes serious complications and seldom requires additional postoperative interventions [8, 9]. The aim of this study is to study the safety and hypotensive effect of trabeculotomy augmented by postoperative medical treatment in patients with open-angle glaucoma and to compare with trabeculectomy augmented by mitomycin C.

2. Patients and methods

In a non-randomized consecutive case series, we studied 82 patients with open-angle glaucoma who underwent trabeculotomy augmented by postoperative medical therapy or trabeculectomy augmented with mitomycin C. A diagnosis of glaucoma was on the gonioscopic finding along with appearance of the optic nerve head cupping and visual alteration according to the guideline of Japan Glaucoma Society [10]. Excluded were patients with angle-closure glaucoma or posttraumatic, uveitic, neovascular, or dysgenetic glaucoma, as well as patients undergoing previous ocular surgery. Before March, 2010, all patients underwent trabeculectomy augmented with mitomycin C, and after April, 2010, all patients underwent trabeculotomy followed by latanoprost 0.004% (Xalatan™, Pfizer, New York, NY, USA), timolol maleate XE 0.5% (Timoptol XE 0.5%™, Santen, Osaka, Japan), and brinzolamide 1% (Azopt™, Alcon, Fort Worth, TX, USA). Patients were followed up for 12 months and the success rate based on intraocular pressure was compared. The study protocol and consent forms were approved by the Human Subjects Committee. When both eyes were eligible, the right eye became the study eye.

3. Surgical procedure

Trabeculectomy: All surgeries were performed by a single surgeon. A modified Cairns-type technique was performed [1]. After making a fornix-based conjunctival flap and dissecting a limbus-based 4 x 4-mm scleral flap, mitomycin C 0.04%-soaked sponges were placed underneath the conjunctival flap for 3 minutes. Afterward, 250 ml of balanced salt solution (Balanced Salt Solution Plus™; Alcon, Fort Worth, TX, USA) was used to wash the surgical area. Paracentesis was carried out followed by a peripheral iridectomy. A scleral flap was sutured with 10/0 nylon, and a conjunctival flap was also sutured with 10/0 nylon with wing stretch technique.

If the bleb was flat or the intraocular pressure was not low enough, laser suture lysis was carried out. If the bleb became flat or localized, needling with angled V-lance was carried out.

Trabeculotomy: After making a fornix-based conjunctival flap, a 4 x 4-mm 4/5 thickness limbus-based scleral flap was created. The outer wall of the Schlemm's canal was incised and removed. The Nagata's semicircular trabeculotome probe was inserted into the Schlemm's canal, and an ocular viscoelastic device (Healon 1%™, Abbott Medical Optics, Santana, CA, USA) was filled in the anterior chamber to reduce postoperative hyphema. The trabeculotome was in-rotated to disrupt the inner wall of the canal, and the viscoelastic material was manually replaced with balanced salt solution. The scleral flap was then sutured watertight with seven 10/0 nylon sutures.

4. Evaluation of outcomes

All patients underwent a detailed ophthalmic examination, including Humphrey visual field analysis and gonioscopy. Patient progress was reviewed at 1 and 3 days; 1 and 2 weeks; and 1, 2, 3, 4, 5, 6, 9, and 12 months after surgery, and intraocular pressure was studied. Intraocular pressure was measured with a Goldman applanation tonometer. Three measurements were recorded in each eye, the mean of which was used in the calculations, with an interval of 2 weeks before surgery at the same time (±1:00). Postoperatively, intraocular pressure was measured at the same time (±1:00) as at baseline. The optic nerve was examined with a

Goldman three-mirror lens and measurements were taken of the size of the disk, the vertical and horizontal cup/disk ratios, the presence of rim notching or splinter hemorrhage, and the presence of peripapillary atrophy. Visual field testing with a Humphrey visual field analyzer (Humphrey-Zeiss, Dublin, CA, USA), Program 30-2 SITA STNADARD™ testing was carried out before surgery and at 6 and 12 months after surgery. Best-corrected visual acuity was measured at the 1-, 2-, 3-, 4-, 5-, 6-, 9-, and 12-month visits, and the logarithm of the minimum angle of resolution (logMAR) was calculated and used for all statistical analyses.

The presence of complications was determined intraoperatively and at every postoperative visit. Hypotony was defined as an intraocular pressure of less than 4 mm Hg after surgery. A shallow anterior chamber was defined as reported by Teehasaenee and Ritch [11]. An intra-ocular pressure spike was defined as an intraocular pressure on the first postoperative day of greater than or equal to 3 mm Hg higher than the preoperative level.

The surgery was considered as a success with an intraocular pressure between 6 and 20 mm Hg and an intraocular pressure reduction of greater than or equal to 30% without additional surgery, compared to the preoperative level with medical therapy. A failure was defined when an eye required further glaucoma surgery or lost visual function.

In case of postoperative intraocular pressure measurements of greater than 21 mm Hg in the trabculectomy group, despite all procedures including laser suture lysis, 5-fluorouracil injection, and needling, intraocular pressure-lowering medication was added. In case of complications requiring surgery or still inadequate intraocular pressure control in both groups, additional procedures could be performed as required.

Study End. All patients were meant to reach a 12-month follow-up, but the following were considered as endpoints: (1) the need for any further surgical procedure (except laser suture lysis, 5-fluorouracil injection, and needling); (2) an intraocular pressure of greater than 21 mm Hg on two consecutive visits; and (3) patient failure to attend scheduled visits, allowing for a margin of tolerance. If the study was ended before month 12, the last values obtained in the trial were considered as the final data.

5. Statistical analysis

The sample size was chosen to assure a power of at least 90% in detecting at least a 2-mm Hg difference between groups with a standard deviation of 2 mm Hg with a two-sided α error of 5%.

Evaluation of continuous variables was achieved using the Student's t-test. To evaluate the difference in intraocular pressures between follow-up intervals, the paired t-test was used. All t-tests were two-tailed. Categoric variables were evaluated with the chi-square test, the Fisher exact test, or the Spearman rank correlation as appropriate. A level of $P < 0.05$ was accepted as statistically significant. Each potential confounding variable was screened for association with the outcome. Only those confounding variables that were statistically associated were eligible to be incorporated into the potential final multivariate model.

For the pairing of groups, age, sex, best-corrected visual acuity, and intraocular pressure at baseline were used for matching. We studied a correlation between the paired observations. If observations were correlated, the F-test was used to study two population variances.

Because a representation of mean intraocular pressure over time could be misleading because of exclusion of cases after failure, the mean intraocular pressure was recalculated by carrying forward the last intraocular pressure reading before repeat surgery. The proportion of surgical failures and adverse events in each treatment group was compared. Success was evaluated on the basis of Kaplan-Meier cumulative probability (log rank test).

6. Results

Table 1 shows the demographics of the patients. Forty-two patients underwent trabeculotomy followed by latanoprost 0.004%, timolol XE 0.5%, and brinzolamide 1%, and 40 patients underwent trabeculectomy augmented with mitomycin C.

	Trabeculotomy augmented by postoperative medication group	Trabeculectomy group	P
Number of patients	42	40	
Age (years)	63.3 ± 9.7 (38 - 78)	67.2 ± 8.2 (41 - 81)	0.1
Gender	24 men, 18 women	18 men, 22 women	0.3
Best-corrected visual acuity	0.681 (0.02 – 1.0)	0.752 (0.1 – 1.0)	-
LogMAR best-corrected visual acuity	0.166±0.338	0.124±0.195	0.3
HFA30-2 MD (dB)	-15.55 ± 6.32 (-26.33 - -4.91)	-16.20 ± 5.10 (-27.48 - -4.88)	0.7
Intraocular pressure (mmHg)	27.9 ± 5.4 (23 – 46)	28.3 ± 4.2 (23 – 42)	0.7
Number of anti- glaucomatous drugs	3.1 ± 0.7 (2 to 4)	3.2 ± 0.7 (2 to 4)	0.9

LogMAR : Log of the minimum angle of resolution

HFA 30-2 MD: Humphrey visual field analyzer Program 30-2 Mean deviation

Parenthesis indicates a range.

Table 1. Demographics of Patients

Mean baseline intraocular pressure was 27.9 ± 5.4 mm Hg in the trabeculotomy group and 28.3 ± 4.2 mm Hg in the trabeculectomy group (P = 0.7). Mean postoperative intraocular pressure was 15.1 ± 2.1 mm Hg at 3 months, 14.7 ± 2.1 mm Hg at 6 months, and 14.9 ± 2.0 mm Hg at 12 months in the trabeculotomy group, and it was 12.2 ± 1.9 mm Hg at 3 months, 12.8 ± 3.0 mm Hg at 6 months, and 13.9 ± 4.2 mm Hg at 12 months in the trabeculectomy group (Figure 1, Table 2). Mean intraocular pressure in the trabeculotomy group was significantly higher than that in the trabeculectomy group at 3 and 6 months (P < 0.0001 at 3 months; P = 0.0005 at 6 months), and there was no significant difference between the groups at 12 months (P = 0.1). At 12 months, 42 patients (100 %) in the trabeculotomy group and 37 patients (92.5 %) in the trabeculectomy group achieved an intraocular pressure of less than or equal to 20 mm Hg and a minimum of 30 percent reduction (P = 0.1) (Figure 2, Table 3).

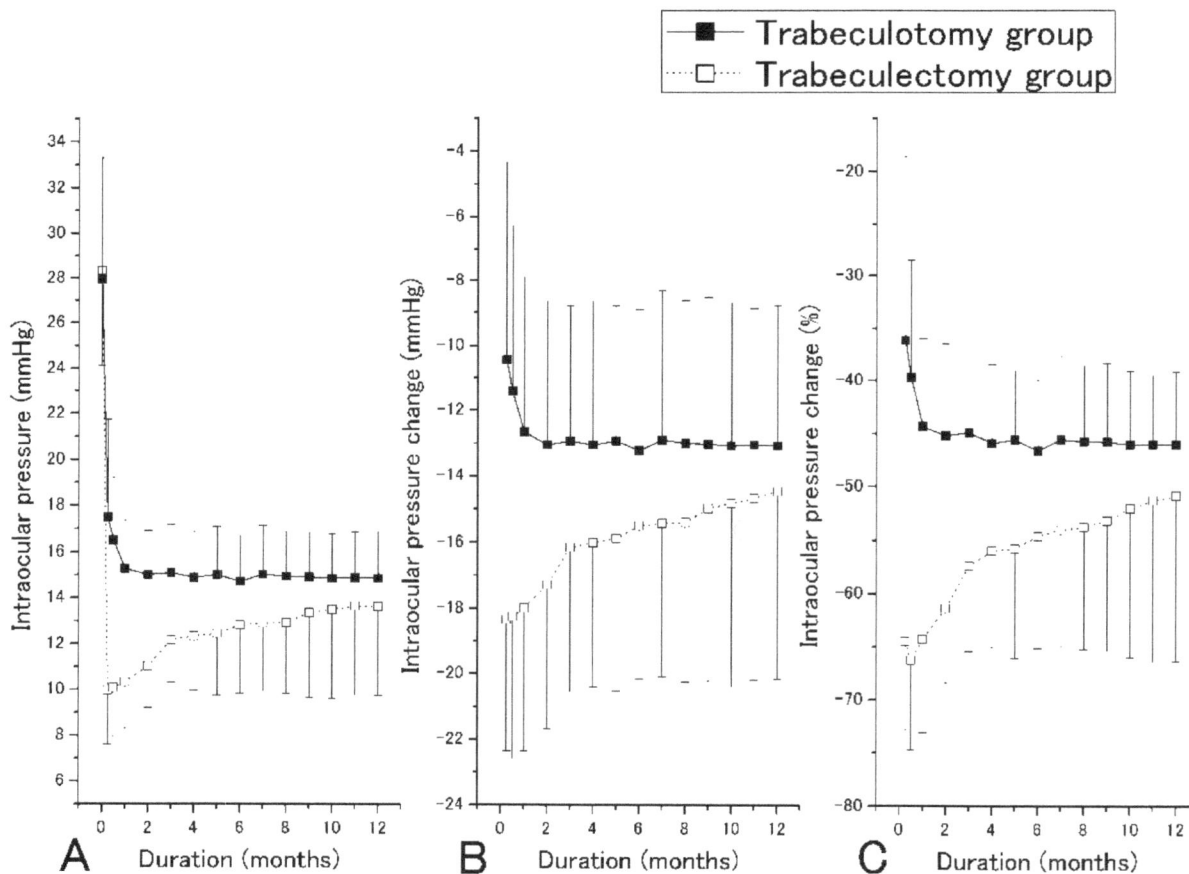

Figure 1. Trabeculotomy

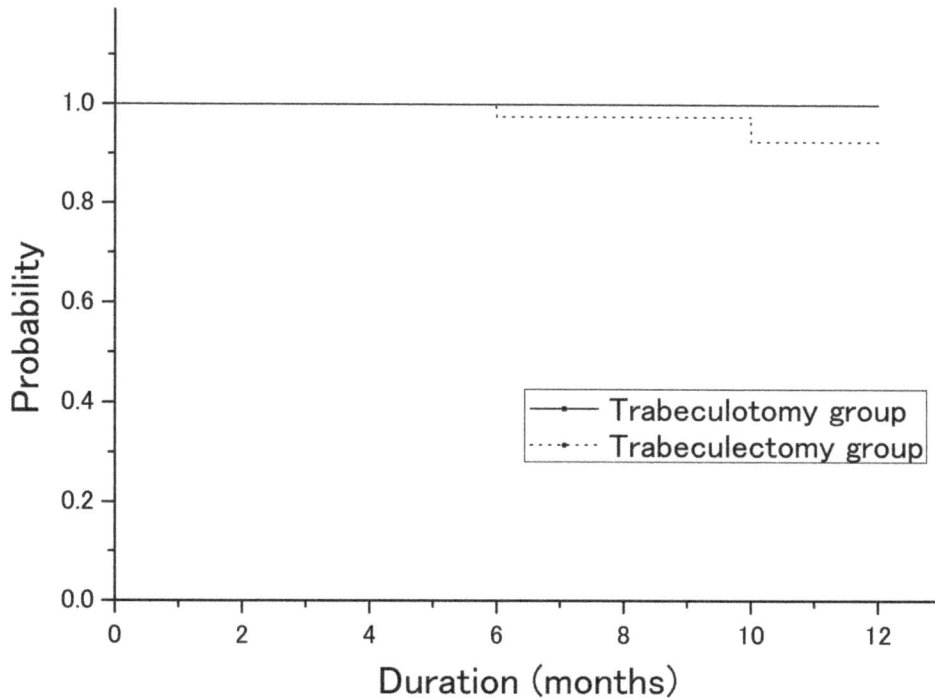

Figure 2. Trabeculotomy

	Trabeculotomy augmented by postoperative medication group	Trabeculectomy group	P
Intraocular pressure (mmHg)			
Baseline	27.9 ± 5.4 (23 – 46)	28.3 ± 4.2 (23 – 42)	0.7
1 month	15.1 ±2.1 (11 – 20)	10.3 ± 2.0 (8 – 17)	<0.0001
3 months	15.1 ±2.1 (11 – 20)	12.2 ± 1.9 (8 – 23)	<0.0001
6 months	14.7 ± 2.1 (12 – 20)	12.8 ± 3.0 (8 - 23)	0.0005
9 months	14.9 ± 1.9 (12 – 18)	13.4 ± 3.7 (8 - 24)	0.0113
12 months	14.9 ± 2.0 (12 – 20)	13.9 ± 4.2 (8 – 25)	0.1
Intraocular pressure (mmHg)			
1 month	-12.7 ± 4.7 (-28 - -8)	-18.0 ± 4.4 (-31 - -11)	<0.0001
3 months	-12.9 ± 4.1 (-26 - -8)	-16.2 ± 4.5 (-31 - -10)	0.0008
6 months	-13.2 ± 4.3 (-28 - -9)	-15.5 ± 4.9 (-30 - -5)	0.0335
9 months	-13.0 ± 4.5 (-28 - -7)	-15.0 ±5.0 (-30 - -5)	0.1
12 months	-13.1 ± 4.3 (-28 - -8)	-14.5 ± 5.3 (-30 - -3)	0.2
Intraocular pressure (%)			
1 month	-44.3 ± 8.4 (-65.8 - -28.6)	-64.4 ± 8.0 (-80.6 - -44.0)	<0.0001
3 months	-44.9 ± 8.7 (-65.8 - -28.6)	-57.2 ± 8.5 (-73.8 - -41.7)	<0.0001

6 months	-46.6 ± 6.7	-54.4 ± 11.3	0.0003
	(-63.2 - -36.0)	(-71.4 - -17.9)	
9 months	-45.8 ± 7.4	-53.0 ± 12.7	0.0023
	(-60.9 - -29.2)	(-71.4 - -17.9)	
12 months	-46.1 ± 6.9	-51.0 ± 14.4	0.1
	(-60.9 - -33.3)	(-71.4 - -10.7)	

Parenthesis indicates a range.

Table 2. Intraocular pressure change

	Trabeculotomy augmented by postoperative medication group	Trabeculectomy group	P
Baseline			
Intraocular pressure	27.9 ± 5.4 (23 – 46)	28.3 ± 4.2 (23 – 42)	0.7
Number of anti-glaucomatous medication	3.1 ± 0.7 (2 to 4)	3.2 ± 0.7 (2 to 4)	0.9
At 12 months			
Intraocular pressure	14.9 ± 2.0 (12 – 20)	13.9 ± 4.2 (8 – 25)	0.1
Success	42 (100.0 %)	37 (92.5 %)	0.1
Failure	0 (0 %)	3 (7.5 %)	
<16 mmHg	37 (84.0 %)	33 (82.5 %)	0.5
<12 mmHg	8 (19.0 %)	23 (57.5 %)	0.0211
Number of anti-glaucomatous medications	3.0 ± 0.0 (3)	0.5 ± 0.9 (0 - 3)	<0.0001

Parenthesis indicates a range.

Table 3. Surgical outcome at 12 months

7. Relationship between intraocular pressure before surgery and at 12 months after surgery

Figure 3 shows the relationship between intraocular pressure before surgery and 12 months after surgery. In both groups, there was a significant increase in the intraocular pressure reduction in relation to an increase in preoperative intraocular pressure (mm Hg: P < 0.0001 in both groups; %: P < 0.0001 in the trabeculotomy group, P = 0.1 in the trabeculectomy group). In the trabeculotomy group, patients with higher preoperative intraocular pressure showed a significantly higher intraocular pressure at 12 months postoperatively (P < 0.0001), although there was no significant correlation between them in the trabeculectomy group (P = 0.2) (Figure 3). At 12 months, 8 eyes (19.0 %) in the trabeculotomy group and 23 eyes (57.5 %) in the trabeculectomy group achieved an intraocular pressure of less than or equal to 12 mm Hg, and there was a significant difference between the two groups (P = 0.0211) (Table 3).

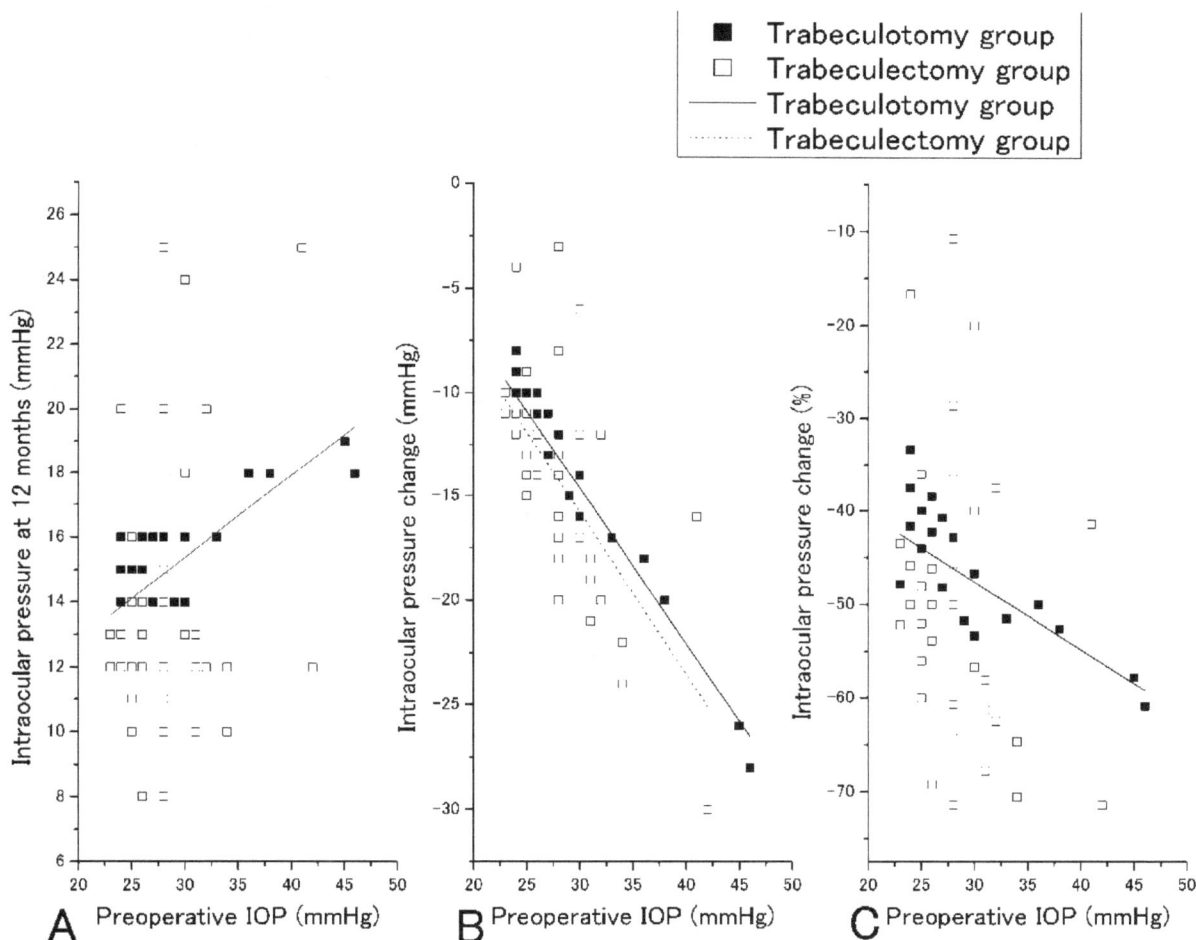

Figure 3. Trabeculotomy

8. Postoperative intraocular pressure-lowering procedures

In the trabeculectomy group, 15 patients (37.5 %) received laser suture lysis, 6 patients (15.0 %) underwent needling procedure, and 3 patients (7.5 %) underwent additional surgery, although no patients in the trabeculotomy group received any postoperative intervention except for topical medical treatment (Table 4).

	Trabeculotomy augmented by postoperative medication group	Trabeculectomy group	P
Number of patients	42	40	
Topical medication	42 (100.0%)	8 (20.0%)	0.0023
Laser suture lysis	0 (0%)	15 (37.5%)	< 0.0001
Needling	0 (0%)	6 (15.0%)	0.0091
5-fluorouracil injection	0 (0%)	0 (0%)	-
Additional surgery	0 (0%)	3 (7.5%)	0.1

Table 4. Postoperative intraocular pressure-lowering procedure

9. Incidence of complications and adverse events

Complications are listed in Table 5. In the trabeculectomy group, 5 eyes (12.5 %) exhibited hypotony and flat/shallow anterior chamber. In the trabeculotomy group, hyphema was observed in 14 eyes (33.3 %) and intraocular pressure spike in 3 eyes (7.1 %). All the bleeding disappeared within one week. No progression of cataract was found in the two groups.

	Trabeculotomy augmented by postoperative medication group	Trabeculectomy group	P
Hypotension	0 (0%)	5 (12.5%)	0.0181
Shallow/flat anterior chamber	0 (0%)	5 (12.5%)	0.0181
Choroidal detachment	0 (0%)	1 (2.5%)	0.3
Intraocular pressure spike	3 (7.1%)	0 (0%)	0.1
Hyphaema	14 (33.3%)	2 (5.0%)	0.0012
Flat bleb	-	5 (12.5%)	-
Anterior iris synechia	0 (0%)	0 (0%)	-
Posterior iris synechia	0 (0%)	0 (0%)	--
Progression of cataract	0 (0%)	0 (0%)	-
Blebitis/endophthalmitis	0 (0%)	0 (0%)	-

Table 5. Incidence of complications

10. Discussion

There was no significant difference in hypotensive efficacy between patients undergoing trabeculotomy augmented by postoperative topical medication and those undergoing trabeculectomy augmented by mitomycin C at 12 months postoperatively. In the current study, 42 eyes (100 %) in the trabeculotomy group and 37 eyes (92.5%) in the trabeculectomy group were considered to be a success defined as an intraocular pressure of less than or equal to 20 mm Hg and a minimum of 30 percent reduction. There was no significant difference in the success rate or intraocular pressure between the trabeculotomy group and the trabeculectomy group at 12 months although the intraocular pressure was higher in the trabeculotomy group at every visit after surgery.

Each surgery had its own advantage. In the trabeculotomy group, all patients showed an intraocular pressure of less than or equal to 20 mm Hg at 12 months. However, patients with higher preoperative pressure showed a relatively higher intraocular pressure at 12 months even though it was less than 20 mm Hg. There was a significant increase in the intraocular pressure at 12 months in relation to the increase in preoperative intraocular pressure. Postoperative intraocular pressure was calculated from the preoperative intraocular pressure by using a correlation equation as follows:

[Intraocular pressure at 12 months] = 0.26 x [preoperative intraocular pressure] + 7.71 (r^2=0.440, P < 0.0001).

Patients receiving trabeculotomy experienced less postoperative surgical interventions than those receiving trabeculectomy. In addition, 3 patients in the trabeculectomy group underwent additional surgery although no patient in the trabeculotomy group did.

In contrast to the trabeculotomy group, there was no significant correlation between preoperative intraocular pressure and postoperative intraocular pressure in patients undergoing trabeculectomy augmented by mitomycin C. This procedure can be employed in all patients to achieve lower postoperative pressure regardless of how high the preoperative intraocular pressure might be. At 12 months, there was a significantly larger percent of eyes of less than or equal to 12 mm Hg in patients undergoing trabeculectomy compared with trabeculotomy despite of postoperative medications. Several investigators have demonstrated that it was pivotal to set a target pressure and achieve it based on patients' visual function [12-15]. Patients with greater visual function deterioration need lower target pressures to maintain residual visual function. According to the target pressure, indication for each of these methodologies should be carefully considered prior to any surgical interventions.

This study has important limitations. The sample size of this study was small, therefore not powered to detect small differences. The small sample size also precluded assessment of safety. Furthermore, a masked study design could have reduced observer bias. The postoperative follow-up period also was short, and therefore we could not assess long-term efficacy and safety.

Although the sample size in each group was small, the current study demonstrated that (1) there was no significant difference in hypotensive efficacy between patients undergoing trabeculotomy augmented by postoperative topical medications and those undergoing trabeculectomy augmented by mitomycin C at 12 months postoperatively and (2) in those receiving trabeculotomy, patients with higher preoperative pressure showed a significantly higher intraocular pressure at 12 months even though less than 20 mm Hg. Future study of a large population is needed to verify these observations. However, this information may be clinically valuable when treating patients with open-angle glaucoma.

Author details

Hiroshi Kobayashi*

Address all correspondence to: kobi@earth.ocn.ne.jp

Department of Ophthalmology, Kanmon Medical Center, Shimonoseki, Japan

No Financial support has been received by any authors and none of the authors has any proprietary interest in the subject matter presented.

References

[1] Cairns DE. Trabeculectomy – a preliminary report of a new method. Am J Ophthalmol 1968;66:673-679.

[2] Lehmann OJ, Bunce C, Matheson MM, Maurino V, et al. Risk factors for development of post-trabeculectomy endophthalmitis. Br J Ophthalmol 2000;84:1349-1353.

[3] Poulsen EJ, Allingham RR. Characteristics and risk factors of infections after glaucoma filtering surgery. J Glaucoma 2000;9:438-443.

[4] DeBry PW, Perkins TW, Heatley G, Kaufman P, et al. Incidence of late-onset bleb-related complications following trabeculectomy with mitomycin. Arch Ophthalmol 2002;120:297-300.

[5] Rothman RF, Liebmann, Ritch R. Low-dose 5-fluorouracil trabeculectomy as initial surgery in uncomplicated glaucoma: long-term follow-up. Ophthalmology 2000;107:1184-1190.

[6] Shigeeda T, Tomidokoro A, Chen YN, Shirato S et al. Long-term follow-up of initial trabeculectomy with mitomycin C for primary open-angle glaucoma in Japanese patients. J Glaucoma 2006;15:195-199.

[7] Tanihara H, Negi A, Akimoto M, Terauchi H et al. Surgical effects of trabeculotomy ab externo on adult eyes with primary open angle glaucoma and pseudoexfoliation syndrome. Arch Ophthalmol 1993;111:1653-1661.

[8] Grehn F. The value of trabeculotomy in glaucoma surgery. Curr Opin Ophthalmol 1995;6:52-60.

[9] Chihara E, Nishida A, Kodo M, Yoshimura N et al. Trabeculotomy ab externo: an alternative treatment in adult patients with primary open-angle glaucoma. Ophthalmic Surg 1993; 24:735-739.

[10] The Japan Glaucoma Society guidelines of glaucoma (3rd edition). Nippon Ganka Gakkai Zasshi 2012;116:387-425.

[11] Teehasaenee C, Ritch R. The use of PhEA 34c in trabeculectomy. Ophthalmology 1986;93:487-490.

[12] Palmberg P. How clinical trial results are changing our thinking about target pressures. Curr Opin Ophthalmol 2002;13:85-88.

[13] Chen PP. Correlation of visual progression between eyes in patients with open-angle glaucoma. Ophthalmology 2002;109:2093-2099.

[14] Palmberg P. Evidence-based target pressures: how to choose and achieve them. Int Ophthalmol Clin 2004;20:393-400.

[15] Aoyama A, Ishida K, Sawada A, Yamamoto T. Target intraocular pressure for stability of visual field loss progression in normal-tension glaucoma. Jpn J Ophthalomol 2010;54:117-123.

8

Refractive Surgery for Myopia

Dieudonne Kaimbo Wa Kaimbo

Abstract

This chapter describes current surgical techniques used to correct myopia, including laser correction (laser surgeries), incisional techniques, intrastromal corneal rings, phakic intraocular lenses, and refractive lensectomy. Contents are based on recent findings published in the medical literature and reflect the most advanced achievements in current refractive surgery for myopia. The chapter presents relevant information that patients, students, optometrists, orthoptists, ophthalmologists, as well as scientists involved in management of myopia need to know about this important topic.

Keywords: Myopia, Refractive Surgery, Correction, Laser correction, Photorefractive keratectomy, LASIK, Phakic intraocular lenses, Refractive lensectomy

1. Introduction

Myopia is the most common eye disease and is one of the leading causes of vision impairment worldwide [124]. Prevalence of myopia is significantly different among racial groups, although its worldwide prevalence is approximately 30% (3–84%) [41]. The highest prevalence is found in East Asia, such as in mainland China [41]. The prevalence of myopia in the US population was estimated in the early 1970s to be 25% in persons aged 12–54 years [111]. A meta-analysis of population-based studies found a prevalence of 25% in persons over age 40 [61]. The World Health Organization has grouped myopia and uncorrected refractive error among the leading causes of blindness and vision impairment in the world [45].

Myopia (nearsightedness) is a refractive error, in which the eye possesses too much optical power (too much plus powers) for its axial length ; as a consequence, images of distant objects focus in front of the retina, when accommodation relaxed (www.checdocs.org).

Myopia has been recognized as a distinct visual disability for millennia and has been known for more than 2000 years, first described by the ancient Greeks [54]. It was probably the ancient

Greeks who coined the term, using the roots *myein* (to close) and *ops* (eye) to characterize those individuals who narrow their eyelids to improve distance visual acuity, the pinhole effect. The focus of distant parallel rays of light falls anterior to the retinal plane and produces a blurred image in myopia. This situation can arise because either the primary refractive components are too powerful or the globe is too long. Thus, myopia can be due to increased corneal or lenticular curvature, or an increase in the lens index of refraction, as occurs with the development of nuclear sclerosis. More commonly, myopia is the result of axial elongation of the posterior segment of the eye.

Myopia is categorized into two groups: (1) low-to-moderate myopia (≤ 6.0 D myoptic spherical equivalent (SE) with or without astigmatism) and (2) high myopia (≥ 6.0 D of myopic SE with or without astigmatism (www.medpagetoday.com).

Low-to-moderate myopia, known as physiologic myopia, is generally defined as that state in which the eye is rendered myopic by a combination of its components of refraction. In this situation, the refractive power of the eye (corneal power plus lens power slightly modified by anterior chamber depth (ACD)) and the axial length are such that its posterior focal plane lies anterior to the retina. Each component has a value within its normal curve of distribution. These eyes demonstrate normal anatomy and physiology. Whether the absence of correlation among the elements of refraction occurs by chance or is a heritable trait is unknown at present. Low-to-moderate myopia is also considered as low-to-moderate refractive errors defined as myopia less than 6.0 diopters (D).

High myopia, also known pathologic, degenerative or malignant myopia, is related to an eye with an axial length exceeding 25.5 or 26 mm, a refractive error of at least -5.0 D and characteristic degenerative changes (eachers%20stangov.uk).

Posterior pole abnormalities typical of high myopia include tessellated fundus, lacquer cracks, diffuse atrophy, patchy atrophy, choroidal neovascularization (CNV), macular atrophy, posterior staphyloma but also straightened and stretched vessels, temporal peripapillary atrophic crescent, hemorrhages, and tilting of the optic disk [48, 52]. Recently, high myopia has been defined as a SE refractive error of at least −6 D associated with characteristic degenerative changes which are more seen in eyes with myopic SE exceeding 8 D.

As elongation of the globe is a key feature of pathological myopia, an axial length of ≥26.5 mm has been adopted as a biometric definition in clinical trials [122], with recent studies reporting a mean of 29 mm (range 26.8–31.5 mm) [129, 130]. Limit of 25.5 mm of myopic eye has been arbitrary fixed as 25, 25.5, or 26.5 mm [74] with an inferior limit of −6 to −10 D of refractive error, providing a cornea of +43.5 D as average refractive power, in the absence of spherophakia or nuclear cataract (eachers%20stangov.uk).

Of greater interest is the determination of the best cutoff for high myopia. Criteria for high myopia that have been used in previous studies include −5.0, −6.0, −10.0, and −12.0 D and there is no universal definition for high myopia [85, 132]. It is thought that at this level, the risks of secondary complications, such as retinal detachment and glaucoma may increase [103, 117, 132]. There may also be further deteriorations in visual field, central visual acuity, increased risks of irregular astigmatism, keratoconus, and peripheral visual field defects.

Most cases of myopia are in children of school age and young adults. The etiology of myopia is not clear, but there is evidence that genetic and environmental factors play a role. The chief complaint is difficult reading at a distance. The diagnosis is made by measurement of refractive errors by refraction [106].

The various modes of treatment of myopia(commonly used methods for correcting myopia) include medical therapy options and surgical therapy options (known as refractive surgery).

2. Medical therapy options

Medical therapy options include eyeglasses (spectacles), contact lenses, and observation. Individuals with asymptomatic myopia may not need eyeglass correction except for activities such as driving or school work. Eyeglasses are the simplest and safest means of correcting myopia; therefore, eyeglasses should be considered before contact lenses or refractive surgery [12]. Contact lenses are used for many reasons. Contact lenses provide better, large field of vision, a greater comfort, and an improved quality of vision. Only contact lenses can give optimal visual function in some conditions such as high myopia, symptomatic anisometropia, aniseikonia, irregular corneal surface, or shape. Further, contact lenses are beneficial in managing unilateral myopia, and some special occupational needs (www.rutzeneye.com).

Spectacles and contact lenses are conservative optical methods. They each have functional limitations such as the problems encountered in wearing spectacles when showering or playing sports, such as individuals involved in certain sports and hazardous activities in which there is risk of eye trauma. Carrying contact lenses solutions and storage solutions can be inconvenient, and wearing contact lenses can increase the risk of corneal infection [106].

3. Surgical therapy options or surgical procedures (refractive surgery)

The term refractive surgery describes various elective procedures that modify the refractive status of the eye [11]. The most commonly used methods for correcting myopia are spectacle correction and contact lens wear. These conservative optical methods provide temporary correction of myopia and remain the first choice, but refractive surgery is increasing significantly. There are a variety of reasons why patients with myopia request refractive surgery as an alternative to contact lenses or spectacles.

These reasons may include the following [28]: (1) contact lenses may be inconvenient, not tolerated, or may be deemed unsafe; (2) spectacles may be associated with unacceptable aberrations, glare, and/or reduction of visual field, and (3) spectacles may be cosmetically unacceptable or inconvenient.

Surgical procedures have been developed in an attempt to permanently correct myopia.

The goal of refractive surgery is to correct myopia by decreasing the refractive power of the eye and to obtain a safe, predictable, stable desired refractive state new optical problems. The refractive power of the eye is reduced, by augmenting the anterior radius of curvature of the cornea (flattening the curvature of the anterior corneal surface) or by insertion of an appropriate synthetic intraocular lens (IOL). Several surgical techniques are available for the treatment of myopia (www.medpagetoday.com).

Several effective options for laser refractive surgery are available to patients, which provide the opportunity to meet more of the needs of an individual patient. These techniques are divided into two groups: those involving surgery on the cornea (corneal refractive surgery) and those involving surgery on the lens (lenticular refractive surgery). Procedures that involve altering the cornea are collectively referred to as keratorefractive surgery, refractive keratoplasty, or refractive corneal surgery [28].

4. Corneal refractive surgery

Corneal refractive procedures used to correct myopia include excimer laser refractive surgery and corneal addition procedures.

Excimer laser refractive surgery for myopia works by removing corneal stroma to lessen the refractive power of the cornea and to bring the image of a viewed object into focus onto the retina rather than in front of it. Corneal addition procedures work by inserting ring segments, a donor lenticule or hydrogel lens inside the cornea, or using compression sutures to steepen the cornea.

4.1. Corneal ablation by excimer laser

This procedure includes lamellar procedures, such as LASIK, and procedures involving surface ablation:

- Laser-assisted stromal in situ keratomileusis (LASIK)

- Photorefractive keratectomy (PRK)

- Laser-assisted subepithelial keratomileusis (LASEK)

- Epithelial laser-assisted in situ keratomileusis (Epi-LASIK)

This is divided into two main procedure groups: surface treatments and flap treatments.

In surface treatments, the skin on the surface of the cornea is removed by physical scraping or peeling and the laser is applied to the surface of the stroma. The laser corrects myopia in modifying the shape of the corneal stroma. In PRK, the surface skin is left to heal naturally with the aid of a contact lens; in laser epithelial keratomileusis (LASEK) or epipolis (Greak for surface) LASIK, known as EpiLASIK, the removed dead skin is replaced and acts like a bandage, while new skin regenerates below it [106].

Flap treatment, called laser-assisted in situ keratomileusis (LASIK), employs a blade or a femtosecond laser to cut a thin flap on the surface of the cornea. The flap is peeled back, and the excimer laser is applied within the body of the cornea stroma. At the end of the procedure, the flap is replaced. A variant of LASIK in sub-Bowman's keratomileusis (SBK), also referred to as "thin-flap LASIK", which differs from LASIK only in that the thickness of the flap is less [106].

4.2. Laser-asssisted stromal in situ keratomileusis (LASIK)

LASIK has become the single most common elective operation with over 35 million procedures performed worldwide by 2010 [1, 97]. Brilliant ideas with bioengineering accomplishments have led to correct about 90% of refractive errors in about a 10-min process with a less discomfort, a recovery time of a few hours and dramatic visual results overnight. www.londonvisionclinic.com)

The concept that refractive error could be corrected by sculpting corneal stromal tissue to change corneal curvature was the brainchild of Jose Ignacio Barraquer Moner in 1948 [24, 26, 27]. Barraquer developed a procedure he coined "keratomileusis" [25], which involved resecting a disc of anterior corneal tissue that was then frozen in liquid nitrogen, placed on a modified watchmaker's lathe, and milled to change corneal curvature. The word "keratomileusis," which is derived from the Greek roots *keras* (hornlike = cornea) and *smileusis* (carving), literally means "sculpting" of the "cornea" [97].

LASIK, the most common procedure for corneal refractive surgery to correct myopia [33, 114], combines lamellar corneal surgery with the accuracy of the excimer laser.

After immobilization of the eye by the positioning of a succion ring, a partial-thickness lamellar corneal flap is cut using a microkeratome (with an oscillating blade to shave 100–200 μm corneal flap, ranging in size from 9 to 10.5 mm); the excimer laser ablation is then performed after the flap to expose the corneal stroma; the laser is then focused and centered over the pupil with the patient looking at affixation light and a preprogrammed excimer ablation of the stroma is performed. The flap is after reflected onto the treated corneal stromal bed [19].

One of the critical steps in this procedure is creation of the corneal flap. Traditionally, the flap was created using mechanical microkeratomes, but during the last few years there has been the emergence of the new ultrashort-pulse lasers (picosecond and femtosecond) [66, 77, 114, 125]. There have been a number of technological advancements to overcome the difficulties associated with intraoperative flap and microkeratome-related complications [33]. The femtosecond laser is one such technology. Current clinical applications of femtosecond lasers have been developed to create flaps for LASIK [59, 96]. The femtosecond laser is a focusable infrared (1053 nm) laser; it employs ultrafast pulses in the 100-fs (100×10^{-15}-s) duration range and makes closely spaced spots which are focused at a preset depth to photodisrupt tissue within the corneal stroma without inflammation and collateral tissue damage. Each laser pulse generates a small amount of microplasma, which results in microscopic gas bubbles in the interface and creates the flap. During treatment, the cornea is flattened with a suction applanating lens to immobilize the eye and to allow treatment of a geometrically simpler planar cornea [77]. Adjacent pulses are scanned across the cornea in a controlled pattern without causing significant inflammation or damage to the surrounding tissue, which possibly results in safer and more predictable flaps [125, 66].

The femtosecond laser was developed as a replacement of the microkeratome; it permits surgeons to customize and create a partial-thickness lamellar corneal flap and customize its diameter within the corneal stroma, providing more accuracy in flap thickness than with previous methods.

4.2.1. Advantages of the femtosecond laser vs mechanical microkeratomes

- Unlike mechanical microkeratomes, which can have variable flap thickness, the femtosecond laser minimizes irregular flap thickness and epithelial injury as it etches a lamellar flap at a desired corneal depth.

- Potential biomechanical and histopathological advantages with femtosecond laser flap creation.

In LASIK, a larger flap is desired (up to 9 or 10 mm in diameter), in high myopes and in patients with large pupils to compensate for any decentration.

With the femtosecond laser, a smaller flap is possible if centered over the optical zone.

- the femtosecond laser has been reported to minimize aberrations and to be less dependent on corneal curvature;

4.2.2. Disadvantages

- increased cost,

- surgical time,

- risk of diffuse lamellar keratitis which is reduced with intensive perioperative topical corticosteroids [19, 33].

In recent studies, outcomes of a femtosecond laser for LASIK (IntraLase, IntraLase Corp., Irvine, CA) [29, 40, 62, 118;] demonstrated more predictable flap thickness, an insignificant increase in higher-order aberrations (HOAs) after flap creation, better uncorrected visual acuity (UCVA), and decreased epithelial injury relative to mechanical microkeratomes. The refractive outcomes after uncomplicated LASIK are relatively stable several years after surgery. The flap perimeter and interface undergo slow wound healing, which allows for early and stable refractive corrections [33, 101]. Although standard laser treatment eliminates conventional refractive errors, it can induce new HOAs that adversely affect the postoperative quality of vision, especially with respect to deterioration of the contrast functions [32, 81, 128]. A clinical refraction, composed of sphere, cylinder, and axis, describes what we now call lower-order aberrations. There exist other types of optical aberrations in the visual pathway of the eye, such as coma and spherical aberration, collectively called higher order. Change in the corneal shape after LASIK toward an oblate pattern is believed to be responsible for inducing spherical aberrations and HOAs after refractive surgery [15, 30].

Aspheric ablation profiles are designed to minimize further inducing spherical aberration by precompensating for its induction or by aiming to maintain the original Q value of the cornea. Wavefront-optimized LASIK compensates specifically for the induced spherical aberration by increasing the pulse energy in the periphery, with good reported visual outcomes [16, 33, 46, 94], and minimization of induced HOA. However, aspheric ablation profiles are not designed to decrease preoperative HOAs. Wavefront-guided ablation profiles are designed to customize the ablation pattern centered on the individual aberration profile of each eye to eliminate the preexisting HOAs and avoid inducing more aberrations. Limitation of such customized treatments in terms of induced changes in corneal asphericity and spherical aberration has been previously reported [30, 33]. There are contradicting reports comparing the results of visual outcome and HOAs between wavefront-guided and aspheric (wavefront-optimized) profiles [33, 43, 65, 69, 75, 82, 88, 100, 112].

4.3. Photorefractive keractectomy (PRK)

PRK is a procedure in which the cornea is reshaped using an excimer laser. PRK evolves epithelial removal and photoablation of Bowman's layer and anterior corneal tissue. In contrast to LASIK, there is no need for flap creation with a microkeratome. PRK can be used in thinner corneas, where creation of a flap may leave less tissue than desired (usually 250 µm of cornea tissue) remaining to the posterior stroma.

PRK was the most commonly performed surgical procedure until the introduction of laser in situ keratomileusis (LASIK) in the mid-1990s. PRK is safe and effective, but the risk of corneal haze, especially in high myopia, is significant. Postoperative pain and slow visual rehabilitation limit the use of PRK (www.jaypeedigital.com).

PRK was first introduced in 1987 [73], and the techniques have continually been modified since then.

The most frequently performed procedures for low-to-moderate myopia utilize the excimer laser, which was first approved for this purpose by the FDA in 1995. A surface ablation technique, PRK was the first procedure performed.

Surgical procedure: An optical zone of 6 mm with a transition zone up to 8 mm is used. The central 6–9 mm of epithelium is removed by one of the several methods: mechanical scraping with a spatula or blade with or without topical alcohol, scraping with an automated brush, using the laser to reduce the thickness and then scrape the residual or to remove epithelium to Bowman's layer, or removing the epithelium with a keratome. The exposed surface is then ablated with laser followed by the placement of a bandage contact lens. A multipass technique is also used for PRK: The total amount of correction is separated into multiple smaller treatments of equal values of sphere and cylinder [91].

The total of these small treatments is equal to the actual-targeted correction. The laser is stopped during 15 s between each pass. All passes are performed during the same surgical procedure. The passes are set so that the operating time at each pass is less than 20 s [91, 92]. Postoperatively, a soft contact lens is inserted on the eye. Corticosteroid drops (fluorometho-lone (FML)) and nonsteroidal anti-inflammatory drugs (ketorolac tromethamine (Acular)) are given every 4 h for the first day and then thrice daily for the next 48 h. Antibiotic drops (ofloxacin 0.3%) are given every 4 h. For myopia more than −6 D, corticosteroids are given twice daily for the first postoperative month, four times daily for the second month, thrice daily for the third month, twice daily for the fourth month, and once daily for the fifth month. Corticosteroids are tapered after the first month follow-up exam. For myopia less than −6 D, corticosteroids are given only during the first week after surgery. Oral analgesics are also prescribed for pain during the first 72 h after surgery [91].

PRK is extremely useful in patients with thin corneas and in patients prone to flap dislocation such as military personnel or contact sports athletes.

Surface ablation techniques compared with LASIK have

4.4. Advantage

More residual posterior corneal stromal tissue is preserved

No stromal flap-related complications.

4.4.1. Disadvantages

More discomfort

Slower recovery of vision (due to the longer re-epithelialization time and potential development of subepithelial haze) [19, 107].

4.4.2. Complications

The corneal wound healing response after PRK is usually more complex than after LASIK for the same amount of correction [76].

- Regression
- Overcorrection and undercorrection
- Haze or corneal scar formation
- Dry eyes
- Infectious keratitis

4.5. Laser-assisted subepithelial keratomileusis

LASEK is indicated in

- low-to-moderate myopia with or without astigmatism
- thin corneas without any signs of keratoconus,
- extreme keratometric values (as in steep or flat corneas),
- deep set eyes and small palpebral fissure,

- recurrent erosion syndrome,

- dry eye,

- glaucoma suspect,

- wide scotopic pupil,

- scleral buckle

LASEK is also indicated in patients and for patients who are prone to trauma, such as military personnel and athletes [116]. Although there is a newer method of creating the epithelial flap mechanically by an epikeratome, without the use of alcohol, LASEK is still considered by many surgeons, for a personal preference or because of the affordability of the mechanical epikeratome.

LASEK involves the creation of an epithelial flap that is put back in position after the laser treatment. Detachment of the epithelial flap is created with placement of a diluted solution of alcohol (typical 15–20%) in a well. Alcohol weakens the adhesions of the basal epithelial cells to the anterior stroma.

4.5.1. Surgical procedure[20, 18, 116]

In brief, after topical anesthesia and lid speculum application, positioning marks are used to mark the corneal surface, and then a semi-sharp circular well is used to administer 18% alcohol for 25–35 s on the corneal epithelial surface [18, 20, 116]. Using vannas scissors and jeweler's forceps, the margins of the delineated area are freed, leaving two to three clock-hours of intact margins for the hinge. Using a Merocel sponge, the loosened epithelium is then peeled back. After standard laser ablation, the epithelial sheet is gently repositioned with the aid of intermittent irrigation. The epithelium is carefully realigned using the preplaced positioning marks and allowed to dry for 3–5 min. Antibiotics and steroids eye drops are given and a bandage contact lens is placed to reduce the mechanical friction by the eyelid and to reduce postoperative pain [8, 91].

4.6. Epithelial laser-assisted in situ keratomileusis (Epi-LASIK)

Epi-LASIK is an innovative new procedure designed to create a thin flap in the epithelium with an epikeratome. Epi-LASIK is also an excellent alternative for patients with thin and steep of flat cornea [84]. The layer is preserved and replaced following the reshaping of the cornea using the excimer laser. Unlike LASER, which uses alcohol to separate the epithelium and the process can kill epithelial cells, Epi-LASEK permits the cells to live and continue to survive following replacement [60]. Preliminary clinical results suggest that Epi-LASEK is a safe and efficient method for the correction of low myopia [14, 83].

4.6.1. Complications

Postoperative dry eye syndrome

Postoperative haze

4.7. Corneal addition procedures

These procedures include the following:

- Intracorneal ring segments (e.g., INTACS); the most commonly used to treat keratoconus.

- Epikeratophakia (removal of epithelium and placement of a donor lenticule of Bowman's layer and anterior stroma). Epikeratophakia (also known as epikeratoplasty and onlay lamellar keratoplasty) was introduced by Werblin et al. It involves removal of the epithelium from the central cornea and preparation of a peripheral annular keratotomy. No microkeratome is used. A lyophilized donor lenticule (consisting of Bowman's layer and anterior stromal) is reconstituted and sewn into the annular keratomy site.

The procedure is used to correct greater degrees of myopia. Complications include irregular astigmatism, delayed visual recovery, and prolonged epithelial defects.

- Keratophakia (intrastromal implantation (insertion) of a donor lenticule of corneal stroma that was previously frozen and reshaped

- Intracorneal lens (implantation of hydrogel lens within the corneal stroma).

- Compression sutures (to modify refractive error by steepening the cornea and reducing astigmatism). Corneal addition procedures, except intracorneal ring segments, are not currently in widespread use (www.medpagetoday.com).

4.8. Corneal relaxation procedures

Radial keratotomy (peripheral deep stromal radial incisions) has been abandoned (www.medpagetoday.com).

RK for myopia involves deep, radial corneal stroma incisions, which weaken the paracentral and peripheral cornea and flatten the central cornea. Patients with low-to-moderate myopia (up to 5 D) achieve the best results with RK in terms of the highest levels of UCVA. Stability of refraction after RK is lower than with many other refractive surgical procedures. The procedure was abandoned because of the long-term complication of bullous keratopathy secondary to endothelial cell loss.

Arcuate keratotomy (paired peripheral stromal incisions parallel to the limbus); the most often used to treat astigmatism after corneal graft surgery.

- Limbal relaxing incisions (deep limbal incisions of varying arc) are used during cataract surgery to reduce preexisting corneal astigmatism. These incisions are a valuable tool for correcting mild astigmatism. There are several nomograms for determining the number and length of peripheral corneal relaxing incisions (PCRIs). For example, www.lricalculator.com features Nichamin and Donnenfeld nomograms; *Cataract and Refractive Surgery* (Kohnen and Koch, 2006) features Koch's nomogram. A PCRI is performed by creating a deep (usually about 600 µm) incision or pair of incisions in the peripheral cornea anterior to the corneal limbus and vascular arcade. The length and placement of the incision(s) depend upon the axis and amount of cylinder. PCRIs work well if the SE is close to plano (due to the coupling effect), and the astigmatism is less than 2.00 D. If necessary, it is possible to add or lengthen a PCRI at a later date. Patients with more significant astigmatism (>2.00 D) typically have greater success with LASIK or PRK than with PCRIs (Focal Point, 2014).

4.8.1. Corneal thermocoagulation

Thermokeratoplasty (heating the peripheral cornea to shrink collagen and steepen the central corneal curvature) can be used to treat hyperopia or presbyopia.

4.9. Criteria for corneal refractive surgery [8, 53]:

Inclusion criteria (10 [53]:

- Age of patient (years): ≥18

- Myopia (up to −12.00 D), with astigmatism, up to 3.00 D

- Refraction with a <0.50 D change of <0.50 D during prior 6 months

- Best correctable visual acuity of >20/20 in both eyes

- No use of soft contact lens use for >7 days before the preoperative visit

- Normal fundus peripheral retina or previously treated with photocoagulation

Informed consent must be obtained from all patients after they receive a detailed description of surgical procedure and a thorough review of its known risks.

To be a candidate for either type of refractive procedure, the patient must have adequate central cornea thickness, regular topography, adequate pupil size, healthy and adequate tear film, and no absolute or relative contraindications to the procedure. LASIK is generally avoided in patients with previous corneal surgery, including PCRIs, in favor of surface ablation. With either procedure, the ablation can be a standard conventional, a wavefront-guided or a wavefront-optimized treatment. Conventional ablation treats lower-order or spherocylindrical aberrations. Wavefront-guided treatment reduces preexisting HOAs and reduces induction of new aberrations by creating a customized ablation profile. Wavefront-optimized ablation provides a customized treatment profile based on the patient's refraction and only treats the HOAs that would be induced by the alteration of this refraction.

Exclusion criteria [8, 53]:

- Age younger than 18 years

- Excessively thin corneas (<500 mm central corneal thickness)

- Topographic evidence of keratoconus [56]

- Eyes with ectatic disorders [99]

- Histories of autoimmune diseases, pregnancy, or current nursing of an infant

- Greater than 2.5 D of difference in sphere and cylinder between eyes

- Previous ocular surgery, corneal diseases, glaucoma, or history of ocular trauma

- Active ocular or systemic disease likely to affect corneal wound healing

4.10. Preoperative evaluation

The preoperative evaluation, a comprehensive medical eye evaluation includes history, examination, diagnosis, and initiation of management (www.rutzeneye.com).

The history should incorporate the elements of the comprehensive medical eye evaluation in order to consider the patient's visual needs and any ocular pathology. In general, a thorough **history may include the following items**:

- Demographic data including name, date of birth, gender, ethnicity, race, occupation, address

- Chief complaint

- History of present ocular disease

- Present status of visual function (e.g., patient's self-assessment of visual status, visual needs, any recent or current ocular symptoms, and use of eyeglasses or contact lenses)

- Ocular history (e.g., prior eye diseases, injuries, surgery, including refractive surgery, or other treatments and medications)

- Systemic history, allergies and adverse reactions to medications,

- Family and social histories: pertinent familial ocular and systemic disease

- Social history such as occupation, smoking history, alcohol use, family and living

- Review of systems

The comprehensive eye examination evaluates an evaluation of the physiologic function and the anatomic status of the eye, visual system, and its related structures. This includes the following elements (www.corneasociety.ca):

- Visual acuity UCVA, with current correction (the power of the present correction recorded) at distance and when appropriate at near

- Measurement of best spectacle-corrected visual acuity (BSCVA) (with refraction when indicated)

- Manifest and cyclogic refractions

- Ocular dominance

- External examination (e.g., lids, lashes, and lacrimal apparatus; orbit; and pertinent facial features)

- Ocular alignment and motility

- Pupillary function; mesopic pupil size measurement using a pupillometer

- Keratometry

- Visual fields by confrontation

- Slit-lamp biomicroscopic examination: eyelid margins and lashes, tear film, conjunctiva, sclera, cornea, anterior chamber, and assessment of peripheral ACD, iris, lens, and anterior vitreous

- Pachymetry

- Corneal topography; computerized videokeratography

- Haze measurement

- Tonometry with Goldmann tonometer

- The fundus ophthalmoscopy: vitreous, retina (including posterior pole and periphery), vasculature, and optic nerve

- Haze measurement

- Assessment of patient's mental and physical status

Anterior segment structures examination includes a close inspection and biomicroscopic evaluation before and after dilation. Posterior segment structures evaluation (examination) requires (needs) a dilated pupil. The peripheral retina examination needs the use of the indirect fundus ophthalmoscopy or slit lamp fundus biomicroscopy. The examination of the macula and optic nerve needs the use of the slit lamp biomicroscope, with diagnostic lenses and OCT.

(www.rutzeneye.com)

The evaluation of myopia requires an assessment of both the refractive status of the eye, the patient's current mode of correction, symptoms, and visual needs. Refraction is often performed in conjunction with a comprehensive medical eye (American Academy of Ophthalmology Preferred. Practice Patterns Committee. Preferred Practice Patterns Guidelines. Comprehensive Adult Medical Eye Evaluation, 2005). Evaluations of myopia include visual acuity, refraction, and refinement. The depth of the corneal lesion can be measured using an optical pachymeter [31]. The combination of manifest refraction, slit-lamp examination, and keratometry is generally sufficient for detecting the most anterior abnormalities.

4.11. Postoperative care

Postoperatively, antibiotics such as tobramycin (Tobrex; Alcon Laboratories, Inc, Fort Worth, Texas, USA), diclofenac 0.1% drops (Basel, Switzerland), and corticosteroids such as dexamethasone 0.1% or prednisolone acetate 1% eyedrops

1. is given four times a day during the first week

2. FML 0.2% is then applied four times daily for four weeks (minimum), based (depending on) on the refraction and IOP;

3.   The drops of FML are tapered gradually three times a day for two weeks and switched to two times a day for two weeks [8]. Lubrication is prescribed as required [91]. After a LASIK, a shield is placed on the eye and taped to the forehead. Patients are instructed to wear their eye shield at night during the week, and not to rub the eyes or swim underwater in order to prevent flap displacement or infectious keratitis.

4.12. Postoperative evaluation [8]

After surgical procedure, the postevaluation includes:

- Measurement of manifest refraction
- Cycloplegic refraction
- UCVA
- BSCVA
- Slit-lamp biomicroscopy
- Dilated funduscopy
- Applanation tonometry
- Corneal topography
- Visual acuity is measured using a standard Snellen acuity chart at 6 m.

Residual stromal bed (RSB) is estimated by two methods: (1) preoperative pachymetry minus predicted flap thickness (according to Pérez-Santonja and associates [86, 87]) minus calculated ablation depth and (2) postoperative pachymetry (using the latest available pachymetry data) minus predicted flap thickness.If enhancement procedures were performed, the RSB is estimated using the sum of the calculated ablation depths for all procedures including the safety and efficacy indexes: Safety = (BCVA postoperative/BCVA preoperative); Efficacy = (UCVA postoperative/BCVA preoperative).

4.13. Results and outcome measures[53, 116]

Primary outcome measures include uncorrected visual accuity, refractive stability, predictability, loss of the best spectacle-corrected visual acuity, aberrometry, contrast sensitivity, and adverse event profile. Evaluation is based on measurement of [53, 116]:

Efficacy measured by the mean postoperative UCVA and the efficacy index, which is the ratio of mean postoperative UCVA to mean preoperative BSCVA.

Predictability measured by the mean postoperative SE within ±0.50 D, and within ±1.00 D of the intended correction; and the percentages of eyes within ±0.50 D and ±1.00 D of emmetropia (target refraction); a lesser likelihood of undercorrection and on the other hand, the more overcorrection seen postoperatively.

Safety measured by lost of two or more lines of BSCVA and the mean postoperative BSCVA; and the safety index, which is the ratio of mean postoperative BSCVA to mean preoperative

BSCVA. The percentage of eyes that lost 1 or more lines of BSCVA at a period of time (six and 12 months) posttreatment [116].

Retreatment and complications percentage of treated eyes retreated for residual myopia and overcorrection.

4.14. LASIK complications [8]

Keratome and flap complications (miscreated flaps, flap striae, interface inflammation, traumatic flap tears with initial flap lift, loss of suction, and epithelial defects, etc.)

Intraoperative complications such as ectasia, flap striae, flap dislocation ;Laser complications such as misinformation/improper ablation, decentered or improperly registered ablation, reduced quality of vision ; complications of healing/infection/inflammation such as recurrent corneal erosions, Infectious keratitis, epithelial ingrowth, diffuse lamellar keratitis (DLK), post-LASIK dry eye syndrome ; other complications of LASIK such as intraocular pressure measurement after LASIK optic neuropathy and glaucoma (www.operationauge.com).

5. Lenticular refractive surgery

Phakic IOLs for the treatment of myopia work by diverging light rays so light rays from a distant object are focused sharply on the retina rather than in front of the retina. Phakic IOLs, therefore, can be inserted in the anterior chamber of the eye in front of the iris or placed in the posterior chamber of the eye behind the iris in front of the natural lens in the ciliary sulcus (www.meddpagetoday.com).

5.1. Refractive lens exchange

This is extraction of the natural lens and insertion of a posterior chamber IOL, that is, "cataract surgery" in the absence of a visually significant cataract.

The technique is a variety of standard cataract surgery. The elements involved are the transparency and softness of the crystalline lens in the absence of cataract and the elongation of the globe, an axial length of ≥26.5 mm associated to high myopia, which in this particular case is the indication for RLE [10].

The ideal technical elements for successful RLE surgery include the following [10]:

- Minimal invasive surgery with minimal trauma to intraocular structures (specially corneal endothelium, iris and other intraocular structures).

- A watertight sub-2.2-mm clear corneal microincision, located optimally less than 1 mm from the limbus on the steepest corneal meridian to minimize surgically induced astigmatism or/ and to reduce preexisting corneal astigmatism [10].

- Capsular bag fixation of an appropriate posterior chamber IOL proven to be associated to a low incidence of posterior capsular pacification (PCO).

Special considerations in cases selected for RLE include the following:

The best approach to RLE surgery includes minimally invasive surgery, through the smallest possible incision.

Specific informed consent for RLE different to different to the one used for cataract surgery must be provided and will include information about potential refractive benefits and complications, and the problem of pseudophakic presbyopia [10].

5.2. Surgical technique [10]

5.2.1. Topical anesthesia

A clear corneal incision and continuous curvilinear capsulorhexis (CCC)

Hydrodissection: cortical cleaving hydrodissection is performed in two separate distal quadrants with decompression of the anterior chamber in order to avoid capsular block syndrome

Prechopping (optional): although the nucleus is not hard in RLE, prechopping facilitates further surgical maneuvers and reduces surgical time

5.2.2. Phacoemulsification

The nucleus is divided based on the technique used: prechopping, chopping, or grooving,

Irrigation/aspiration

An adequate viscoelastic is injected deep in the capsular bag to reform the bag and prepare it for IOL insertion

IOL insertion. After IOL insertion, bimanual

Irrigation/aspiration is performed to remove all viscoelastic material

A preservative-free antibiotic is injected into the anterior chamber, and then the stroma at the incisions is hydrated to assist self-sealing.

5.2.3. Complications

Post-RLE retinal detachment

Cystoid macular edema in the first few weeks after surgery

PCO, which can develop from months to years after the surgical procedure

A decrease in twilight vision (with halo perception and glare) after implantation of multifocal IOLs.

Choroidal neovascular membrane (CNV) formation

Myopic macular degeneration

RLE is indicated in high refractive error in the absence of cataract. RLE, however, is specifically only indicated in presbyopic eye [10]. In general, due to the fact that at present for restoration of near intermediate, and distance vision, multifocal IOLs are at present superior to the available accommodating IOLs. The main challenge involved is to reach emmetropia with rapid recovery using the astigmatically neutral incisions of modern cataract surgery [10].

6. Phakic IOL

This is the insertion of an additional synthetic lens in front of the natural lens, placed either behind the iris in the ciliary sulcus or clipped to the iris in the anterior chamber.

Implantation of IOLs in the phakic eye (phakic intraocular lense, pIOL) is a relatively new technique to correct high ametropia.

pIOLs are used for correcting moderate and high ametropias and allowing maintenance of accommodation while offering good quality of vision, some reversibility of the procedure, and possible management of postoperative error [21, 39, 50, 72, 79, 123]. Among the IOLs are the implantable Collamer lens (ICL, Staar Surgical, Monrovia, CA), a foldable posterior chamber IOL, the veriflex lens (Verflex Phakic IOL), an iris-claw lens with hydrophobic polysiloxane foldable design. Implantation of both types of pIOLs is increasingly popular because it is technically undemanding while offering high predictability and a good safety profile.

Implantation of pIOLs is a reversible refractive procedure, preserving the patient's accommodative function with minimal induction of HOAs compared with corneal photoablative procedures [86].

Corneal ablation surgical procedures such as PRK or LASIK laser are usually the preferred options by refractive surgeons for correcting refractive errors [86]. However, the range of safe dioptric correction for these procedures has been progressively limited due to the mid- and long-term complications observed, particularly in cases of high refractive error, such as keratectasia [95], corneal haze [105], regression [8], dry eye [119], or poor postoperative visual quality [55, 89]. It has been shown that photoablative refractive surgery in high ametropia can lead to a significant increase in ocular aberrations [89] and decrease in visual performance [55]. Furthermore, corneal photoablation has a decreased predictability for the correction of high refractive error because of the unknown and unpredictable effects on corneal biomechanics [98].

Intraocular refractive procedures have become a safe, efficient, and predictable alternative for treating high ametropias when the use of corneal photoablative procedures is not possible or high risk [86].

The progress of intraocular refractive surgery is due to advances made in IOL designs, surgical tools and procedures, and viscoelastic substances, [7].

The advantages of implantation of pIOLs are:

• a reversible refractive procedure and

- a preservation of the accommodative function with

- a minimal induction of HOAs compared with corneal photoablative procedures [86, 102].

pIOLs may be divided into anterior chamber and posterior chamber lenses, with anterior chamber lenses being further divided into angle-supported and iris-fixated [86].

Angle-supported pIOLs were first implanted in 1986. Initial designs induced significant rates of complications (corneal endothelial cell loss, chronic uveitis or pupil ovalization). These lenses have shown good refractive results in the long term [58, 86, 87].

Despite this, as an intraocular procedure, it has potential-associated complications such as cataract, chronic uveitis, pupil ovalization, corneal endothelial cell loss, pigmentary dispersion syndrome, pupillary block glaucoma, astigmatism, or endophthalmitis [34].

6.1. Indications of phakic lenses

Patients with high myopia and who are poor candidates for laser correction.

6.1.1. Criteria

Age: 21–45 years with ACD of 3.0 mm or greater and Shaffer grade II as determined by gonioscopy

Myopia ranging from −3 to −20 D

Astigmatism less than or equal to 2.5 D

Stable refraction (less than 0.5 D change for 6 months)

Clear crystalline lens

Ametropia not suitable, appropriate for excimer laser surgery

Unsatisfactory vision, intolerance of contact lenses, or spectacles

A minimum endothelial cell density

No ocular pathology such as corneal disorders, glaucoma, uveitis, maculopathy

6.1.2. Surgical procedure for anterior chamber angle-supported phakic IOL

Anterior chamber phakic IOL implantation can be performed under typical or peribulbar anesthesia

Pilocarpine is instilled in the eye 30 min before surgery to protect the crystalline lens at the time of IOL implantation

Creating a superior scleral tunnel or a temporal clear corneal incision (2-6.5 mm, of size, according to the IOL model)

The anterior chamber is filled with cohesive viscoelastic

The lens is introduced toward the angle from the incision (the first footplace is inserted in the iridocorneal angle, the second haptic is then placed, avoiding having their folding over the haptic)

The lens is then rotated with a lens dialer to the meridian in which the pupil is best centered in relation to the IOL optic

A peripheral iridectomy is performed

The incision is closed

Removal of the viscoelastic

Topical antibiotics and corticosteroids are applied for times daily for 4–6 weeks

6.1.3. Surgical procedure for iris-fixated phakic IOLs

Preoperative application of topical pilocarpine

Corneal, limbal, or scleral tunnel incision (at least 5.3 or 6.3 mm)

The "claw" haptics are fixated to the iris by enclavation by two side-port incisions at 10 and 2 o'clock

The lens is implanted vertically through the incision, and rotated and centered in front of the pupil with haptics at 3 and 9 o'clock positions

The anterior chamber is filled cohesive OVD material

Watertight wound closure

Removing of the OVD material

Antibiotics and corticosteroids are prescribed for 2–4 weeks.

6.1.4. Surgical technique for posterior chamber phakic IOLs

Topical mydriatics (combination cyclopentolate and phenylephrine), 30 min before surgery

Topical or peribulbar anesthesia

A 2.0–3.0 mm temporal clear corneal tunnel

Placement of cohesive OVD

The posterior chamber IOL is introduced into the anterior chamber

Each footplace is then placed one after the other beneath the iris

Intraoperative iridectomy (or 2 peripheral Nd:YAG laser iridotomis 2 weeks before surgery)

Removing of the OVD material

Acetylcholine chloride is injected

Antibiotics and steroids eyedrops are used three times a day for 1 week with tapered doses for 3 weeks and tropicamide 0.5% two times a day for 2 days.

There are a number of studies evaluating the outcomes obtained with the different models of ICL, and therefore, there is a complete characterization of the refractive outcomes and complications resulting from the implantation of this pIOL [2, 3, 4, 5, 47, 70, 90, 104].

6.2. Preoperative assessment and patient selection for pIOLs implantation [86]

A complete ophthalmological examination is performed before the suy and will include:

- a comprehensive clinical history;

- Visual acuities (uncorrected and best-corrected) visual acuity (using preferably optotypes in logMAR scale under photopic conditions, 85 cd/m^2);

- Refraction (objective, subjective, and cycloplegic);

- Biomicroscopy of anterior segment

- Intraocular pressure measurement (preferably Goldmann tonometry); scotopic pupillometry; corneal topography; biometric analysis (axial length, white-to-white (WTW) distance, and ACD); corneal endothelial analysis by means of a specular microscopy; binocularity evaluation; and fundus evaluation.

The patient must be properly inform about the procedure and risks of the surgery.Spherical hydrophilic contact lenses, toric hydrophilic and rigid gas permeable contact lenses must be discontinued during a period of at least 1week before the preoperative examination, [80]. The refractive error stability during at least 1 year before the intervention must be confirmed. The principal indication for pIOL implantation includes prior contraindication of corneal refractive surgery for myopic or hyperopic refractive error correction (including postsurgical central keratometry below 36 D, RSB of <250 mm or residual central corneal thickness below 400 μm after the programmed laser ablation) [86].

Contraindications of this type of implant for refractive error correction include the following:

Age under 18 years old (except in certain cases of anisometropic amblyopia with intolerance to contact lenses and noncompliance with other less invasive treatment options) [9], previous intraocular surgery, ACD (corneal endothelium-anterior surface of the crystalline lens) <3 mm, glaucoma, history of uveitis, lenticular opacity, nontreated peripheral retinal lesions, scotopic pupillary diameter of >7 mm, neuro-ophthalmological disease, pregnancy or breastfeeding, and unrealistic expectations [17, 57].

Also, any condition associated to a potential zonular weakening and fragility of the ciliary processes should be also considered as a contraindication for the implantation of PRL, such as history of ocular trauma with secondary zonular damage, Marfan' s syndrome diagnosis [42]. A preoperative evaluation of the zonule by means of ultrasound technology is indicated [86].

6.3.1. Results of angle-supported anterior chamber pIOLs [64]

Anterior chamber pIOLs generally demonstrate good predictability, efficacy, and safety. However, there is a tendency toward undercorrection of the refractive error [58, 120].

6.3.2. Results of iris-fixated anterior chamber pIOLs [64]

Several studies with long follow-up demonstrated good predictability, efficacy, and safety of the nontoric and toric pIOL models. With the toric pIOL models, larger amount of preoperative astigmatism can be managed successfully [6, 38, 49, 51, 121].

6.3.3. Results of posterior chamber pIOLs [64]

Visual acuity, predictability, efficacy, and safety of the ICL (Staar Surgical Co.) and the phakic refractive lens (PRL; Carl Zeiss Meditec) posterior chamber pIOL models are good. In a United States Food and Drug Administration (FDA) study, the ICL pIOL showed good functional results with a low complication rate (ICL, 2004). In a prospective study comparing matched populations of laser in situ keratomileusis (LASIK) and Visian ICL implantation, the ICL performed better than LASIK in almost all measures of safety, efficacy, predictability, and stability (Sanders, 2007). In a few case reports, results with the toric posterior chamber pIOL have been shown [63, 64]. Schallhorn et al. [64] report better results with the toric ICL than with conventional PRK in a randomized prospective comparison of safety, efficacy, predictability, and stability. In summary, pIOLs show good refractive and clinical results. They demonstrate reversibility, high optical quality, potential gain in visual acuity in myopic patients due to retinal magnification, and correction is not limited by corneal thickness or topography. With proper anatomical conditions (especially sufficient ACD), pIOLs also show good refractive and clinical results in hyperopic patients [22]. Phakic IOLs preserve corneal architecture, asphericity, and accommodation. With recent innovations in the design of toric pIOLs, spherocylindrical correction is also feasible. However, pIOL implantation is not without complications. The spectrum of common and rare complications with each type of pIOL is presented in the following section.

6.4. Complications

6.4.1. General complications of intraocular surgery [64]

With the increasing use of topical or parabulbar anesthesia, complications due to anesthesia such as retrobulbar hemorrhage, penetration of the globe, or life-threatening systemic side effects from accidental injection into the optic nerve are very rare.

Because implantation of a pIOL is an intraocular procedure, it bears a potential risk for the development of postoperative endophthalmitis. The risk for this complication in general cataract surgery with implantation of a posterior chamber IOL is 0.1–0.7% with an optimal antiseptic perioperative treatment regimen.

6.4.2. Complications of angle-supported anterior chamber pIOL

Loss of corneal endothelial cells

Pupil ovalization/iris retraction

Optical quality, glare, halos

Surgically induced astigmatism

Pigment dispersion or IOL deposits

Chronic inflammation or uveitis

Intraocular pressure elevation/pupillary block glaucoma

pIOL rotation

Cataractogenesis

Retinal detachment

Oddities

6.4.3. Complications of iris-fixated anterior chamber pIOL

Optical quality, glare, halos

Surgically induced astigmatism

Loss of corneal endothelial cells

Pigment dispersion/lens deposits

Intraocular pressure elevation

pIOL rotation

Cataractogenesis

Retinal detachment

Oddities

6.4.4. Complications of posterior chamber pIOL

Complications for the ICL and PRL are similar and are related to the position of the pIOL between the rear surface of the iris and the front surface of the crystalline lens. Complications such as cataractogenesis, pupillary bloc, and glaucoma are due to pIOL design materials (www.ecavolunteer.org).

Optical quality, glare, halos

Surgically induced astigmatism

Loss of corneal endothelial cells

Pigment dispersion/IOL deposits/intraocular pressure elevation

Chronic inflammation/uveitis

Pupil ovalization/iris retraction

Pupillary block/malignant glaucoma

Decentration/incorrect size/pIOL rotation

Cataractogenesis

Retinal detachment

Oddity: zonular dehiscence

7. Multifocal lens

These lenses have concentric ring segments that have two different focal lengths for distance and near vision.

7.1. Toric lens

These lenses have a cylindrical power to address astigmatism.

8. Conclusion

The prevalence of refractive errors is high, affecting approximately one-third of persons 40 years or older in the United States and Western Europe. Myopia is the most common eye disease and is one of the leading causes of vision impairment.

This chapter describes current surgical techniques used to correct myopia, including laser correction (laser surgeries), incisional techniques, intrastromal corneal rings, pIOLs, and refractive lensectomy.

Spectacles and contact lenses remain the first choice for correcting refractive error, but refractive surgery, especially LASIK, is increasing significantly.

There are now several surgical techniques available for the treatment of myopia. The excimer laser, and pIOLs and RLE are promising tools for refractive surgery. The techniques are still developing, and it is certain that there will be significant advances in the future.

Author details

Dieudonne Kaimbo Wa Kaimbo*

Address all correspondence to: dieudonne_kaimbo@yahoo.com

University of Kinshasa, Kinshasa, Congo (DRC)

References

[1] 2010 Comprehensive Report of the Global Refractive Surgery Market. *Market Scope*, 2011:10–11.

[2] Alfonso JF, Ferna´ndez-Vega L, Lisa C, Fernandes P, Gonza´lez-Me´ijome JM, Monte´s-Mico´ R. Collagen copolymer toric posterior chamber phakic intraocular lens in eyes with keratoconus. *J Cataract Refract Surg* 2010b; 36:906–916.

[3] Alfonso JF, Lisa C, Abdelhamid A, Fernandes P, Jorge J, Monte´s-Mico´ R. Three-year follow-up of subjective vault following myopic implantable Collamer lens implantation. *Graefes Arch Clin Exp Ophthalmol* 2010a; 248:1827–1835.

[4] Alfonso JF, Lisa C, Abdelhamid A, Monte´s-Mico´ R, Poo- Lo´pez A, Ferrer-Blasco T. Posterior chamber phakic intraocular lenses after penetrating keratoplasty. *J Cataract Refract Surg* 2009; 35:1166–1173.

[5] Alfonso JF, Palacios A, Monte´s-Mico´ R. Myopic phakic STAAR Collamer posterior chamber intraocular lenses for keratoconus. *J Refract Surg* 2008; 24:867–874.

[6] Alio JL, Mulet ME, Guti_errez R, Galal A. Artisan toric phakic intraocular lens for correction of astigmatism. *J Refract Surg* 2005; 21:324–331.

[7] Alio JL. Advances in phakic intraocular lenses: indications, efficacy, safety, and new designs. *Curr Opin Ophthalmol* 2004;15:350–357.

[8] Alio´ JL, Muftuoglu O, Ortiz D, Pe´rez-Santonja JJ, Artola A, Ayala MJ, et al. Ten-year follow-up of laser in situ keratomileusis for high myopia. *Am J Ophthalmol* 2008; 145:55–64.

[9] Alio´ JL, Toffaha BT, Laria C, Pin~ero DP. Phakic intraocular lens implantation for treatment of anisometropia and amblyopia in children: 5-year follow-up. *J Refract Surg* 2011; 1:1–8.

[10] Alió JL, Andrzej Grzybowski A, Aswad AEI, Dorota Romaniuk D. Refractive lens exchange. *Survey Ophthalmol* 2014;59:579–598.

[11] American Academy of Ophthalmology Preferred. Practice Patterns Committee. Preferred Practice Patterns Guidelines. Comprehensive Adult Medical Eye Evaluation, San Francisco, CA: America Academy of Ophthalmology, 2005.

[12] American Academy of Ophthalmology. Refractive Management/Intervention Panel refractive Errors & refractive surgery, San Francisco, CA. American Academy of Ophthalmology, 2007. Available at: http://www.aao.org/ppp.

[13] American Academy of Ophthalmology. Basic and Clinical Science Course. Section 3. Optics, Refraction, and Contact Lenses, San Francisco, CA. American Academy of Ophthalmology, 2010–2011.

[14] Anderson NJ, Beran RF, Schneider TL. Epi-LASEK for the correction of myopia and myopic astigmatism. *J Cataract Refract Surg* 2002;28:1343–1347.

[15] Anera RG, Jimenez JR, Jimenez del Barco L, Bermudez J, Hita E. Changes in corneal asphericity after laser in situ keratomileusis. *J Cataract Refract Surg* 2003;29:762–768. doi:10.1016/S0886-3350(02)01895-3

[16] Arbelaez MC, Vidal C, Arba-Mosquera S. Excimer laser correction of moderate to high astigmatism with a non-wavefront guided aberration-free ablation profile: six-month results. *J Cataract Refract Surg* 2009;35:1789–1798. doi:10.1016/j.jcrs.2009.05.035

[17] Artola A, Jimenez-Alfaro I, Ruiz-Moreno, et al: Proper patient assessment. Selection and preparation, in Alio JL, Perez-Santonja JJ (eds): Refractive Surgery with Phakic IOLs. Fundamentals and Practice. Highlights of Ophthalmology International. El Dorado, Panama, 2004, pp 37–53.

[18] Azar DT, Ang RT. Laser subepithelial keratomileusis: evolution of alcohol assisted flap surface ablation. *Int Ophthalmol Clin* 2002;42:89–97.

[19] Azar DT, Chang J-H, Han KY. Wound healing after keratorefractive surgery: review of biological and optical considerations. *Cornea* 2012; 31(01):S9–S19. doi:10.1097/ICO.0b013e31826ab0a7.

[20] Azar DT, Taneri S, Chen CC. Laser subepithelial keratomileusis (LASEK) review and clinicopathological correlations. *MEJO* 2002;10:54–59.

[21] Baikoff G, Colin J. Intraocular lenses in phakic patients. *Ophthalmol Clin N Am* 1992;5:789–995.

[22] Baikoff G. Anterior segment OCT and phakic intraocular lenses: a perspective. *J Cataract Refract Surg* 2006; 32:1827–1835.

[23] Bains KC, Hamill MB. Refractive enhancement of pseudopakic patient. Focal points, Clinical Module for ophthalmologists. *Am Acad Ophthalmol* 2014;32(11).

[24] Barraquer JL. Autokeratoplasty with optical carving for the correction of myopia (keratomileusis) (Spanish). *An Med Espec* 1965;51(1):66–82.

[25] Barraquer JL. Keratomileusis. *Int Surg* 1967;48(2):103–117.

[26] Barraquer JL. Method for cutting lamellar grafts in frozen cornea. New orientation for refractive surgery. *Arch Soc Am Oftal Optom* 1958;1:271–286.

[27] Barraquer JL. Queratoplastia refractive. *EstudiosbebInformaciones Oftalmológicas* 1949;10:2–21.

[28] Barsam A, Allan BDS. Excimer laser refractive surgery versus phakic intraocular lenses for the correction of moderate to high myopia (Review). *The Cochrane Library* 2014, Issue 6. Copyright © 2014 The Cochrane Collaboration. Published by John Wiley & Sons, Ltd.

[29] Binder PS. Flap dimensions created with the IntraLase FS laser. *J Cataract Refract Surg* 2004;30(1):26–32.

[30] Bottos KM, Leite MT, Aventura-Isidro M, et al. Corneal asphericity and spherical aberration after refractive surgery. *J Cataract Refract Surg* 2011;37:1109–1115. doi: 10.1016/j.jcrs.2010.12.058

[31] Campos M, Wang XW, Hertzog L, Lee M, Clapham T, Trokel SL, McDonnell PJ. Ablation rates and surface of 193 nm excimer laser keratectomies. Invest Ophthalmol Vis Sci 1993; 34(8):2493-2500.

[32] Chalita MR, Chavala S, Xu M, Krueger RR. Wavefront analysis in post-LASIK Eyes and its correlation with visual symptoms, refraction, and topography. *Ophthalmology* 2004;111:447–453. doi:10.1016/j.ophtha.2003.06.022.

[33] Chen S, Feng Y, Stojanovic A, Jankov MR, Wang Q. IntraLase femtosecond laser vs mechanical microkeratomes in LASIK for myopia: a systematic review and meta-analysis. *J Refract Surg* 2012;28 (1):15–24.doi: 10.3928/1081597X-20111228-02

[34] Comaish IF, Lawless MA. Phakic intraocular lenses. *Curr Opin Ophthalmol* 2002; 13:7–13.

[35] Comaish IF, Lawless MA. Progressive post-LASIK keratectasia: biomechanical instability or chronic disease process? *J Cataract Refract Surg* 2002;28:2206-2213.

[36] Curtin B, Karlin D. Axial length measurements and fundus changes of the myopic eye. *Am J Ophthalmol* 1971;71:42–53.

[37] Dart J. Extended-wear contact lenses, microbial keratitis, and public health. *Lancet* 1999; 354(9174):174–175.

[38] Dick HB, Ali_o J, Bianchetti M, Budo C, Christiaans BJ, El- Danasoury MA, Güell JL, Krumeich J, Landesz M, Loureiro F, Luyten GPM, Marinho A, Rahhal MS, Schwenn O, Spirig R, Thomann U, Venter J. Toric phakic intraocular lens; European multicenter study. *Ophthalmology* 2003; 110:150–162.

[39] Dick HB, Tehrani M, Aliyeva S. Contrast sensitivity after implantation of toric iris-claw lenses in phakic eyes. *J Cataract Refract Surg* 2004;30:2284-2289.

[40] Durrie DS, Kezirian GM. Femtosecond laser versus mechanical keratome flaps in wavefront-guided laser in situ keratomileusis: prospective contralateral eye study. *J Cataract Refract Surg* 2005;31:120-126.

[41] Edwards MH, Lam CS. The epidemiology of myopia in Hong Kong. *Ann Acad Med Sing* 2004; 33:34–38.

[42] Eleftheriadis H, Amoros S, Bilbao R, Teijeiro MA. Spontaneous dislocation of a phakic refractive lens into the vitreous cavity. *J Cataract Refract Surg* 2004; 30:2013–2016.

[43] Feng J, Yu J, Wang Q. Meta-analysis of wavefront-guided vs. wavefront-optimized LASIK for myopia. *Optom Vis Sci.* 2011;88:463–469.

[44] Foulks GN. Prolonging contact lens wear and making contact lens wear safer. *Am J Ophthalmol* 2006;141(2):369–3673.

[45] Fredrick DR. Myopia. *BMJ* 2002;324(7347):1195–1199.

[46] George MR, Shah RA, Hood C, Krueger RR. Transitioning to optimized correction with the Wavelight ALLEGRETTO WAVE: case distribution, visual outcomes and wavefront aberrations. *J Refract Surg* 2010;26:S806–S813. doi: 10.3928/1081597X-20100921-07

[47] Gonvers M, Othenin-Girard P, Bornet C, Sickenberg M. Implantable contact lens for moderate to high myopia: short-term follow-up of 2 models. *J Cataract Refract Surg* 2001; 27: 380–388.

[48] Grossniklaus H, Green W. Pathologic findings in pathologic myopia. *Retina* 1992;12:127–133.

[49] Güell JL, Morral M, Gris O, Gaytan J, Sisquella M, Manero F. Five-year follow-up of 399 phakic Artisan–Verisyse implantation for myopia, hyperopia, and/or astigmatism. *Ophthalmology* 2008; 115:1002–1012.

[50] Güell JL, Vázquez M, Gris O. Adjustable refractive surgery: 60 mm Artisan lens plus laser in situ keratomileusis for the correction of high myopia. *Ophthalmology* 2001;108:945–952.

[51] Güell JL, Vazquez M, Malecaze F, Manero F, Gris O, Velasco F, Hulin H, Pujol J. Artisan toric phakic intraocular lens for the correction of high astigmatism. *Am J Ophthalmol* 2003; 136:442–447.

[52] Hayashi K, Ohno-Matsui K, Shimada N, Moriyama M, Kojima A, Hayashi W, et al. Longterm pattern of progression of myopic maculopathy: a natural history study. *Ophthalmology* 2010; 117: 1595–1611.

[53] He L, Liu A, Manche EE. Wavefront-guided versus wavefront-optimized laser in situ keratomileusis for patients with myopia: a prospective randomized contralateral eye study. *Am J Ophthalmol* 2014;157:1170–1178.

[54] Hirschberg J. *The history of ophthalmology. The middle ages; the sixteenth and seventeenth centuries.* West Germany 1985;2:263–279.

[55] Holladay JT, Dudeja DR, Chang J. Functional vision and corneal changes after laser in situ keratomileusis determined by contrast sensitivity, glare testing, and corneal topography. *JCataract Refract Surg* 1999; 25:663–669.

[56] Holladay JT. Keratoconus detection using corneal topography. *J Refract Surg* 2009;25(10 Suppl):S958–S962.

[57] Hoyos JE, Dementiev DD, Cigales M, Hoyos-Chaco'n J, Hoffer KJ. Phakic refractive lens experience in Spain. *J Cataract Refract Surg* 2002; 28:1939–1946.

[58] Javaloy J, Alio' JL, Iradier MT, Abdelrahman AM, Javaloy T, Borra's F. Outcomes of ZB5M angle-supported anterior chamber phakic intraocular lenses at 12 years. *J Refract Surg* 2007; 23:147–158.

[59] Juhasz T, Loesel FH, Kurtz RM, et al. Corneal refractive surgery with femtosecond lasers. IEEE *J Selected Topics Quantum Electron* 1999;5:902–910.

[60] Katsanevaki VJ, Naoumidi II, Kalyvianaki MI, et al. Epi-LASIK: histological findings of separated epithelial sheets 24 hours after treatment. *J Refract Surg* 2006; 22:151–154.

[61] Kempen JH, Mitchell P, Lee KE, et al. The prevalence of refractive errors among adults in the United States, Western Europe, and Australia. *Arch Ophthalmol* 2004; (122):495–505.

[62] Kezirian GM, Stonecipher KG. Comparison of the IntraLase femtosecond laser and mechanical microkeratomes for laser in situ keratomileusis. *J Cataract Refract Surg* 2004;30:804–811.

[63] Koch DD, Kohnen T, Mamalis N, Obstbaum SA, Rosen ES. Celebrating 10 years. *J Cataract Refract Surg* 2006;32(1):1.

[64] Kohnen T, Kook D, Morral, Güell JL. Phakic intraocular lenses Part 2: Results and complications. *J Cataract Refract Surg* 2010; 36:2168–2194.

[65] Koller T, Iseli HP, Hafezi F, Mrochen M, Seiler T. Q-factor customized ablation profile for the correction of myopic astigmatism. *J Cataract Refract Surg* 2006;32:584–589. doi:10.1016/j.jcrs.2006.01.049

[66] Kurtz RM, Horvath C, Liu HH, et al. Lamellar refractive surgery with scanned intrastromal picosecond and femtosecond laser pulses in animal eyes. *J Refract Surg* 1998;14:541–548.

[67] Lee JB, Kim JS, Choe C, Seong GJ, Kim EK. Comparison of two procedures: photorefractive keratectomy versus laser in situ keratomileusis for low to moderate myopia. *Jap J Ophthalmol* 2001;45(5):487–491.

[68] Lee JB, Seong GJ, Lee JH, et al. Comparison of laser epithelial keratomileusis and photorefractive keratectomy for low to moderate myopia. *J Cataract Refract Surg* 2001;27:565–570.

[69] Myrowitz EH, Chuck RS. A comparison of wavefront-optimized and wavefront-guided ablations. *Curr Opin Ophthalmol.* 2009;20:247–250. doi:10.1097/ICU.0b013e32832a2336

[70] Lovisolo CF, Reinstein DZ. Phakic intraocular lenses. *Surv Ophthalmol* 2005; 50:549–587.

[71] Maldonado BA, Onnis R. Results of laser in situ keratomileusis in different degrees of myopia. *Ophthalmology* 1998; 105:606–611.

[72] Malecaze FJ, Hulin H, Bierer P, et al. A randomized paired eye comparison of two techniques for treating moderately high myopia: LASIK and Artisan phakic lens. *Ophthalmology* 2002;109:1622–1630.

[73] McDonald MB, Frantz JM, Klyce SD, et al. Central photorefractive keratectomy for myopia in the nonhuman primate cornea. *Arch Ophthalmol* 1990; 108:799.

[74] Metge P. Definitions. Vol La myopie forte, *Masson*, Paris, 1994, pp 14–17.

[75] Miraftab M, Seyedian M, Hashemi H. Wavefront-guided vs Wavefront-optimized LASIK: randomized clinical trial comparing contralateral eyes. *J Refract Surg.* 2011;27:245–250. doi:10.3928/1081597X-20100812-02

[76] Mohan RR, Hutcheon AE, Choi R, et al. Apoptosis, necrosis, proliferation, and myofibroblast generation in the stroma following LASIK and PRK. *Exp Eye Res* 2003; 76:71–87.

[77] Montés-Micó R, Rodríguez-Galietero A, Alió JL. Femtosecond laser versus mechanical keratome LASIK for myopia. *Ophthalmology* 2007;114:62–68.

[78] Mutti DO, Zadnik K, Adams AJ. Myopia. The nature versus nurture debate goes on. *Invest Ophthalmo Vis Sci* 1996;37:952-957.

[79] Nio YK, Jansonius NM, Wijdh RH, et al. Effect of methods of myopia correction on visual acuity, contrast sensitivity and depth of focus. *J Cataract Refract Surg* 2003; 29:2082–2095.

[80] Nouruzi H, Rajavi J, Okhovatpour MA. Time to resolution of corneal edema after long-term contact lens wear. *Am J Ophthalmol* 2006; 142:671–673.

[81] Oshika T, Okamoto C, Samejima T, Tokunaga T, Miyata K. Contrast sensitivity function and ocular higher-order wavefront aberrations in normal human eyes. *Ophthalmology*. 2006;113:1807–1812. doi:10.1016/j.ophtha.2006.03.061

[82] Padmanabhan P, Mrochen M, Basuthkar S, Viswanathan D, Joseph R. Wavefront-guided versus wavefront-optimized laser in situ keratomileusis: contralateral comparative study. *J Cataract Refract Surg* 2008;34:389–397. doi:10.1016/j.jcrs.2007.10.028

[83] Pallikaris IG, Kalyvianaki MI, Katsanevaki VJ, Ginis HS. Epi-LASIK : preliminary clinical results of an alternative surface ablation procedure. *J Cataract Refract Surg* 2005;31 (5):879–885.

[84] Pallikaris IG, Katsanevaki VJ, Kalyvianaki MI, et al. Advances in subepithelial excimer refractive surgery techniques: Epi-LASIK. *Curr Opin Ophthalmol* 2003; 14:207–212.

[85] Percival SP. Redefinition of high myopia: the relationship of axial length measurement to myopic pathology and its relevance to cataract surgery. *Dev Ophthalmol* 1987;14:42–46.

[86] Pérez-Cambrodı´RJ, Pinero DP,Ferrer-Blasco T, Cervino A Brautaset R. The posterior chamber phakic refractive lens (PRL): a review. *Eye* 2013; 27:14–21.

[87] Pérez-Santonja JJ, Alio´ JL, Jime´nez-Alfaro I, Zato MA. Surgical correction of severe miopıa with an angle supported phakic intraocular lens. *J Cataract Refract Surg* 2000; 26:1288–1302.

[88] Perez-Straziota CE, Randleman JB, Stulting RD. Visual acuity and higher-order aberrations with wavefront-guided and wavefront-optimized laser in situ keratomileusis. *J Cataract Refract Surg*. 2010;36:437–441. doi:10.1016/j.jcrs.2009.09.031

[89] Pesudovs K. Wavefront aberration outcomes of LASIK for high myopia and high hyperopia. *J Refract Surg* 2005; 21:S508–S512.

[90] Petternel V, Ko°ppl CM, Dejaco-Ruhswurm I, Findl O, Skorpik C, Drexler W. Effect of accommodation and pupil size on the movement of a posterior chamber lens in the phakic eye. *Ophthalmology* 2004; 111:325–331.

[91] Pop M, Payette Y. Photorefractive keratectomy versus laser in situ keratomileusis: a control-matched study. *Ophthalmology* 2000;107:251–257.

[92] Pop M. Prompt re-treatment after photorefractive keratectomy. *J Cataract Refract Surg* 1998;24:320–326.

[93] Pruett R. Pathologic myopia, in Albert DM, Jakobiec JF (eds): Principles and Practice of Ophthalmology. Philadelphia, PA: Saunders Co, 1994, pp 878–889.

[94] Randleman JB, Perez-Straziota CE, Hu MH, et al. Higher-order aberrations after wavefront-optimized photorefractive keratectomy and laser in situ keratomileusis. *J Cataract Refract Surg* 2009;35:260–264. doi:10.1016/j.jcrs.2008.10.032

[95] Randleman JB. Post-laser in-situ keratomileusis ectasia: current understanding and future directions. *Curr Opin Ophthalmol* 2006; 17:406–412.

[96] Ratkay-Traub I, Juhasz T, Horvath C, et al. Ultra-short pulse (femtosecond) laser surgery: initial use in LASIK flap creation. *Ophthalmol Clin N Am* 2001;14:347–355, viii–ix.

[97] Reinstein DZ, Archer TJ, Gobbe M. The history of LASIK. *J Refract Surg* 2012;28:291–298.

[98] Roy AS, Dupps WJ Jr. Effects of altered corneal stiffness on native and postoperative LASIK corneal biomechanical behavior: A whole-eye finite element analysis. *J Refract Surg* 2009; 25:875–887.

[99] Saad A, Gatinel D. Evaluation of total and corneal wavefront high order aberrations for the detection of forme fruste keratoconus. *Invest Ophthalmol Vis Sci* 2012;53(6): 2978–2992.

[100] Sáles CS, Manche EE. One-year outcomes from a prospective, randomized, eye-to-eye comparison of wavefront-guided and wavefront-optimized LASIK in myopes. *Ophthalmology* 2013;120:2396–2402. doi:10.1016/j.ophtha.2013.05.010

[101] Sandoval HP, Castro LEF, Vroman DT, Soloman KD. Refractive Surgery Survey 2004. *J Cataract Refract Surg* 2005;31:221–223. doi:10.1016/j.jcrs.2004.08.047.

[102] Sarver EJ, Sanders DR, Vukich JA. Image quality in myopic eyes corrected with laser in situ keratomileusis and phakic intraocular lens. *J Refract Surg* 2003; 19:397–404.

[103] Saw SM. How blinding is pathological myopia? *Br J Ophthalmol* 2006;90:525–526.

[104] Schmidinger G, Lackner B, Pieh S, Skorpik C. Long-term changes in posterior chamber phakic intraocular Collamer lens vaulting in myopic patients. *Ophthalmology* 2010; 117: 1506–1511.

[105] Shojaei A, Mohammad-Rabei H, Eslani M, Elahi B, Noorizadeh F. Long-term evaluation of complications and results of photorefractive keratectomy in myopia: an 8-year follow-up. *Cornea* 2009; 28:304–310.

[106] Shortt AJ, Allan BD. *Photorefractive keratectomy (PRK) versus laser-assisted in-situ keratomileusis (LASIK) for laser-assisted in-situ keratomileusis (LASIK) versus photorefractive keratectomy (PRK) for myopia (Review) 19* Copyright © 2013 The Cochrane Collaboration. Published by JohnWiley & Sons, Ltd. myopia. *Cochrane Database of Systematic Reviews* 2006, Issue 2. (doi: 10.1002/14651858.CD005135)

[107] Shortt AJ, Allan BD. Photorefractive keratectomy (PRK) versus laser-assisted in-situ keratomileusis (LASIK) for myopia. Cochrane Database Syst Rev 2006CD005135.

[108] Shortt AJ, Bunce C, Allan BD. Evidence for superior efficacy and safety of LASIK over photorefractive keratectomy for correction of myopia. *Ophthalmology* 2006;113:1897–1908.

[109] Silva R. Myopic maculopathy: a review. *Ophthalmologica* 2012;228(4):197–213.

[110] Soubrane G. Choroidal neovascularization in pathologic myopia: recent developments in diagnosis and treatment. *Surv Ophthalmol* 2008;53:121–138.

[111] Sperduto RD, Seigel D, Roberts J, Rowland M. Prevalence of myopia in the United States. *Arch Ophthalmol* 1983;101(3):405–407.

[112] Stonecipher KG, Kezirian GM. Wavefront-optimized versus wavefront-guided LASIK for myopic astigmatism with the ALLEGRETTO WAVE: three-month results of a prospective FDA trial. *J Refract Surg* 2008;24:S424–S431.

[113] Sugar A, Rapuano CJ, Culbertson WW, et al. Laser in situ keratomileusis for myopia and astigmatism: safety and efficacy: a report by the American Academy of Ophthalmology. *Ophthalmology* 2002;109(1):175–187. doi:10.1016/S0161-6420(01)00966-6

[114] Sugar A. Ultrafast (femtosecond) laser refractive surgery. *Curr Opin Ophthalmol* 2002;13(4):246–249. doi:10.1097/00055735-200208000-00011.

[115] Tano Y. Pathologic myopia: where are we now? *Am J Ophthalmol* 2002;134:645–660.

[116] Tobaigy FM, Ghanem RC, Sayegh RR, Hallak JA, Azar DT. A control-matched comparison of laser epithelial keratomileusis and laser in situ keratomileusis for low to moderate myopia. *Am J Ophthalmol* 2006; 142:901–908.

[117] Tong L, Saw SM, Chan ES, Yap M, Lee HY, Kwang YP, Tan D. Screening for myopia and refractive errors using LogMar visual acuity by optometrists and a simplified visual acuity chart by nurses. *Optom Vis Sci* 2004;81(9):684–691.

[118] Tran DB, Sarayba MA, Bor Z, et al. Randomized prospective clinical study comparing induced aberrations with IntraLase and Hansatome flap creation in fellow eyes: potential impact on wavefront-guided laser in situ keratomileusis. *J Cataract Refract Surg* 2005;31:97–105.

[119] Tuisku IS, Lindbohm N, Wilson SE, Tervo TM. Dry eye and corneal sensitivity after high myopic LASIK. *J Refract Surg* 2007; 23:338–342.

[120] Utine CA, Bayraktar S, Kaya V, Eren H, Prente I, Kucuksumer Y, Kevser MA, Yilmaz O F. ZB5M anterior chamber and Fyodorov's posterior chamber phakic intraocular lenses: long-term follow-up. *J Refract Surg* 2006; 22:906–910.

[121] Venter J. Artisan phakic intraocular lens in patients with keratoconus. *J Refract Surg* 2009; 25:759–764.

[122] Verteporfin in Photodynamic Therapy Study Group. Photodynamic therapy of subfoveal choroidal neovascularization in pathologic myopia. 1-year results of a randomized clinical trial-VIP report no. 1. *Ophthalmology* 2001;108:841-852.

[123] Visessook N, Peng Q, Apple D, et al. Pathological examination of an explanted phakic posterior chamber intraocular lens. *J Cataract Refract Surg* 1999;25:216–222.

[124] Vitale S, Sperduto RD, Ferris FL, III. Increased prevalence of myopia in the United States between 1971–1972 and 1999–2004. *Arch Ophthalmol* 2004;127:1632–1639.

[125] Vogel A, Günther T, Asiyo-Vogel M, Birngruber R. Factors determining the refractive effects of intrastromal photorefractive keratectomy with the picosecond laser. *J Cataract Refract Surg* 1997;23(9):1301–1310.

[126] Werblin TP, Kaufman HE, Friedlander MH, Granet N. Epikeratophakia: the surgical correction of aphakia. III. Preliminary results of a prospective clinical trial. *Arch Ophthalmol* 1981;99(11):1957–1960.

[127] Yamamoto I, Rogers AH., Reichel E, Yates PA, Duker JS. Intravitreal bevacizumab (Avastin) as treatment for subfoveal choroidal neovascularization secondary to pathological myopia. *Br J Ophthalmol* 2007;91:157–160.

[128] Yamane N, Miyata K, Samejima T, et al. Ocular higher-order aberrations and contrast sensitivity after conventional laser in situ keratomileusis. *Invest Ophthalmol Vis Sci* 2004;45:3986–3990. doi:10.1167/iovs.04-0629

[129] Yoshida T, Ohno-Matsui K, Ohtake Y, Takashima T, Futagami S, Baba T, Yasuzumi K, Tokoro T, Michizuki M. Long-term visual prognosis of choroidal neovascularization in high myopia: a comparison between age groups. *Ophthalmology* 2002; 109:712–719.

[130] Yoshida T, Ohno-Matsui K, Yasuzumi K, Kojima A, Shimada N, Futagami S, Tokoro T, Mochizuki M. Myopic choroidal neovascularization : a 10-year follow-up. *Ophthalmology* 2003;110:1297–1305.

[131] You QS, Xu L, Yang H, et al. Five-year incidence of visual impairment and blindness in adult. Chinese: the Beijing eye study. *Ophthalmology* 2011;118:1069–1075. *Epub 2011.*

[132] Younan C, Mitchell P, Cumming RG, Rochtchina E, Wang U. Myopia and incident cataract and cataract surgery: the Blue Mountains Eye Study. *Invest Ophthalmol Vis Sci* 2002;43(12):3625–3632.

9

Subconjunctival Mitomycin C Injection into Pterygium Decreases Its Size and Reduces Associated Complications

Mohammad Hossien Davari, Hoda Gheytasi and Esmat Davari

Abstract

Purpose: To evaluate the safety and efficacy of subconjunctival injection of low dose mitomycin C (MMC) in the management of pterygium.

Patients and Methods: This study was carried out from February 2006 to April 2007 in the eye clinic of Vali-e-Asr Hospital of Birjand University of Medical Sciences. Forty eyes with primary pterygia received 0.02 mg MMC (0.1 ml of 0.2 mg/ml solution, Kyowa Hakko Kogyo Co. Ltd., Tokyo, Japan) subconjunctivally injected into the body of the pterygium. Patients were followed at one day, one week, one month, six months and one year after injection. Patients were examined at all visits for conjunctivally erythematic, epithelial defects; intraocular pressure; topography; keratometry; and other complications (complete slit-lamp examinations).

Results: The only complications after subconjunctival MMC injection were mild chemosis, long discomfort, and redness in the site of injection for four days, which were seen in six patients (15%). Toxicity of MMC was not observed in any case. The size of pterygia reduced in 83% of cases and progression were not seen in any case. The amount of astigmatism reduced in 70% cases (mean 0.27 diopter).

Conclusion: Subconjunctival injection of MMC is an effective treatment and allows exact titration of MMC delivery to the activated fibroblasts and minimizes epithelial toxicity but long term follow up is required.

Keywords: pterygium, mitomycin C, subconjunctival, complication

1. Introduction

Pterygium is a fibro vascular overgrowth of degenerative conjunctiva tissue that extends across the limbos and invades the cornea [1, 2].

The risk factors for pterygium development include exposure to ultraviolet (UV) light, dust, wind, heat, dryness, and smoke [2].

The primary indication for surgical removal of pterygium is visual acuity reduction. The cause of this phenomenon is extension of remaining scar to visual axis [3]. Irregular astigmatism, reduced vision, discomfort and irritation, difficulty with contact lens wear, refractive surgery, and cosmetic deformity are other reasons for surgical intervention [3].

A wide range of surgical procedures for removal of pterygia have been reported [4]. However, recurrences after excision have been reported to be very high. For example, it has been reported as high as 30% to 80% with the bare sclera technique [5]. The conjunctiva auto graft transplantation effectively prevents pterygium recurrence [6, 7, 8].

MMC is an antibiotic, antineoplastic agent that selectively inhibits the synthesis of DNA, cellular division, and protein [9]. The mechanism of action of MMC seems to be inhibition of fibroblast proliferation at the level of the episclera [10, 11, 12].The benefit of MMC is having prolonged, but not permanent, effectiveness on suppressing human fibroblasts [13, 14, 15].

Although multiple studies have reported recurrence rates of approximately 5% to 12% with the use of topical MMC [16, 17], this technique has been associated with rare but significant conjunctival and corneal toxicity [16]. In an attempt to decrease ocular morbidity, the intraoperative administration of MMC was applied directly to the sclera bed, which has gained increasing acceptance. Recently, combined pterygium removal with intraoperative MMC and conjunctiva auto grafting for primary and recurrent pterygium has been described [18].

The purpose of this study was to evaluate effectiveness by applying MMC at low concentration and low volume.

2. Patients and methods

Forty consecutive patients (40 eyes) with primary pterygia who attended the eye clinic, Vali-Asr Hospital of Birjand University of Medical Sciences, between 2006 and 2007 were included in this study. All patients had primary pterygium grade I or II and were not previously operated. The grading used was as follows: Grade 1: small primary pterygium, fibrous type, pinguecular, and classical type. Grade II: advanced primary pterygium with no optical zone involvement. Grade III: advanced primary pterygium with optical zone involvement. We selected only grade I and II.

A complete ocular examination, including slit-lamp examination and hematological examination, was performed on each patient. All surgeries were performed by one surgeon (Dr.Davari). Satisfaction of Ethical Clearance Committee accepted and all patients were given an explanation of the procedure and informed consent was obtained from all.

A drop of tetracaine 0.5% was instilled in the involved eye for topical anesthesia and the patients were injected subconjunctivally with a 30-gauge needle on an insulin syringe containing 0.1 ml of 0.2 mg/ml of MMC (Kyowa Hakko Kogyo Co. Ltd. Tokyo, Japan). The injection was done directly into the pterygium 1mm from limbos (Figure 1).

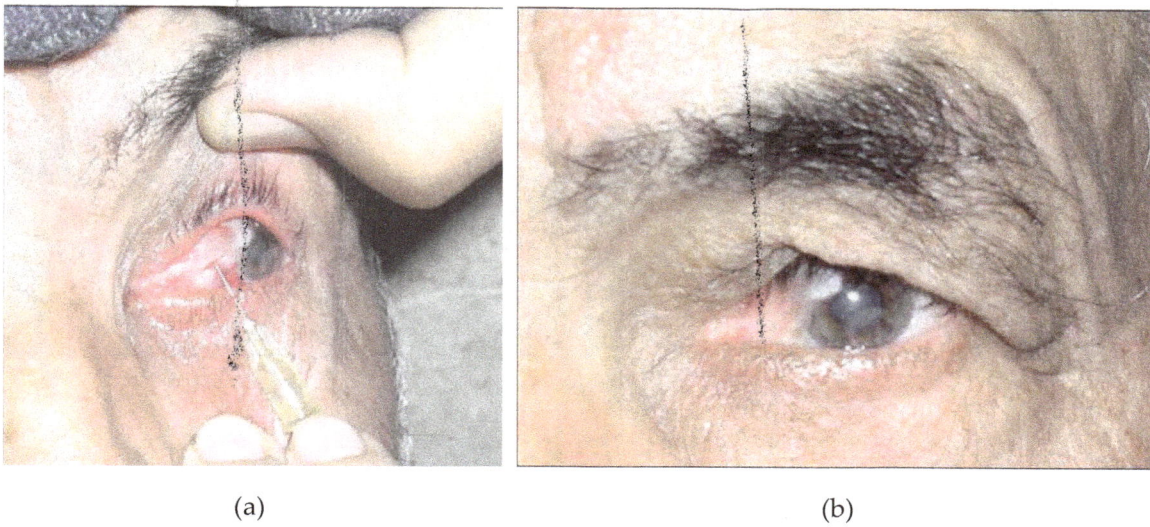

(a)   (b)

Figure 1. (a) Subconjunctival injection of MMC directly into pterygium, (b) After injection of MMC the degree of inflammation reduced.

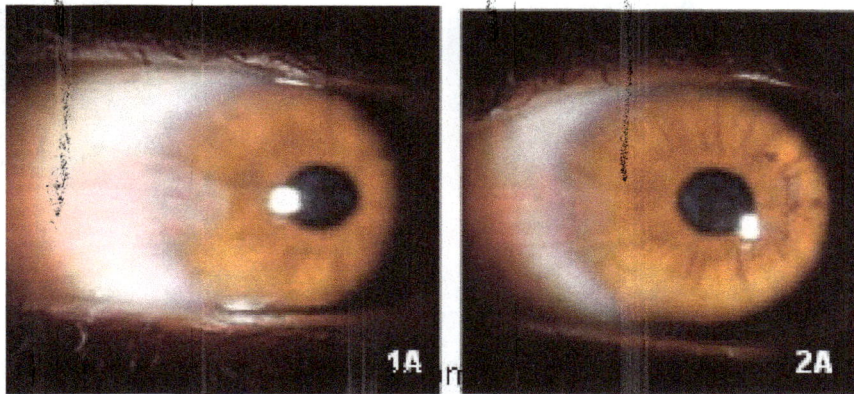

Figure 2. (1A) Before MMC injection, (2A) After MMC injection

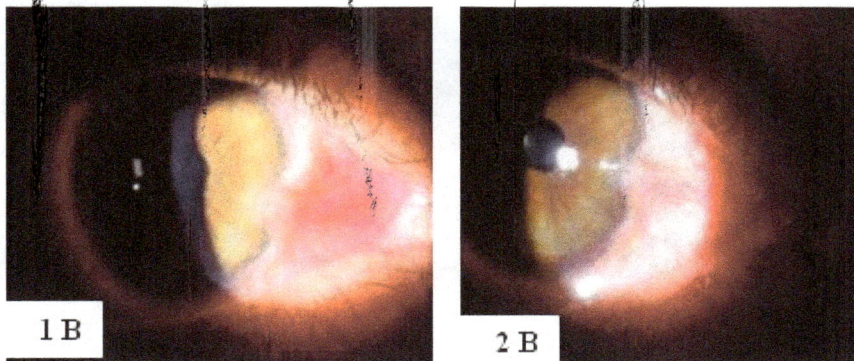

Figure 3. (1B) Before MMC injection, (2B) After MMC injection

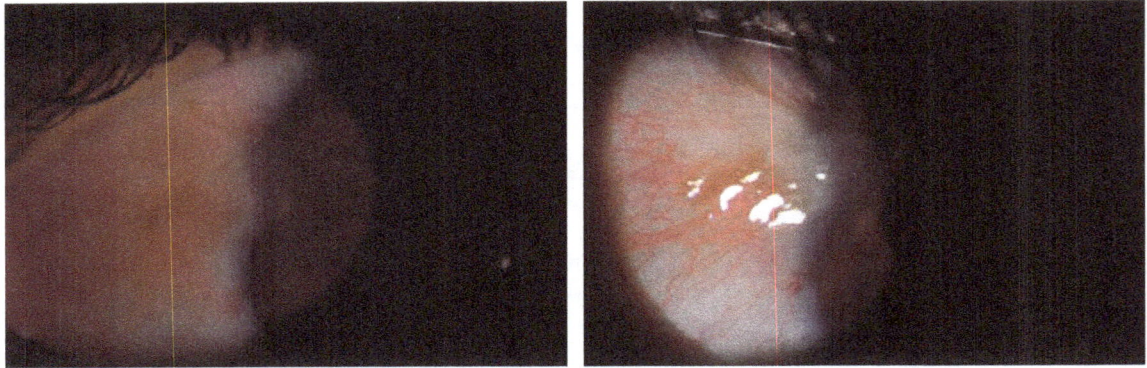

(a)   (b)

Figure 4. (a) Before MMC injection, (b) After MMC injection

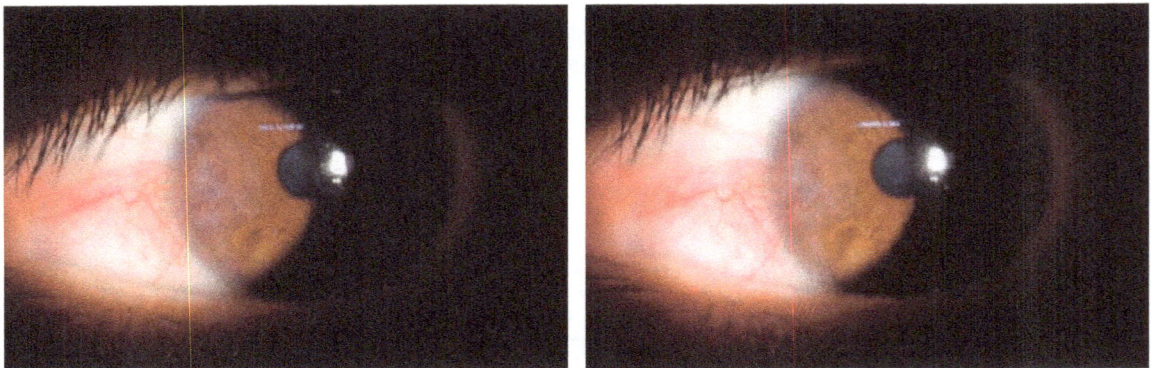

(a)   (b)

Figure 5. (a) Before MMC injection, (b) After MMC injection

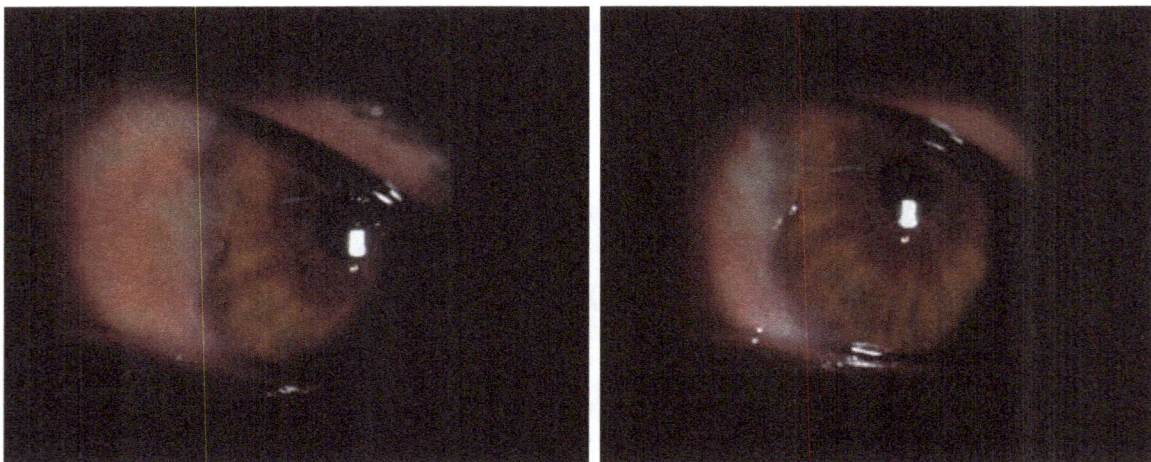

(a)   (b)

Figure 6. (a) Before MMC injection, (b) After MMC injection

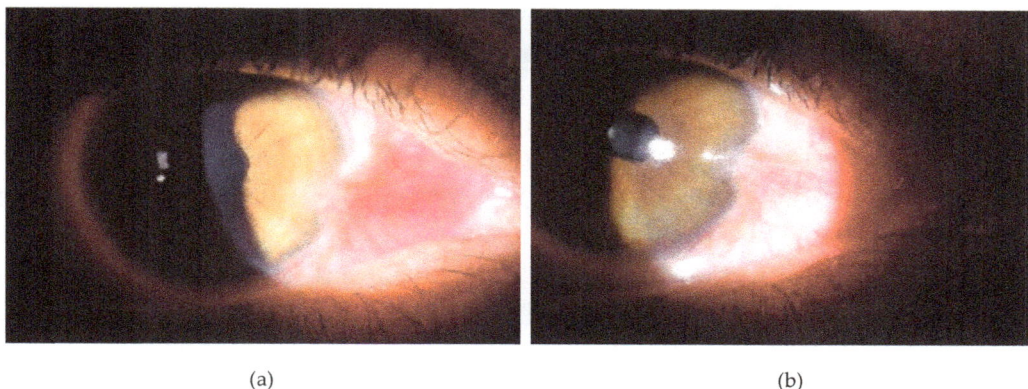

(a)   (b)

Figure 7. (a) Before MMC injection, (b) After MMC injection

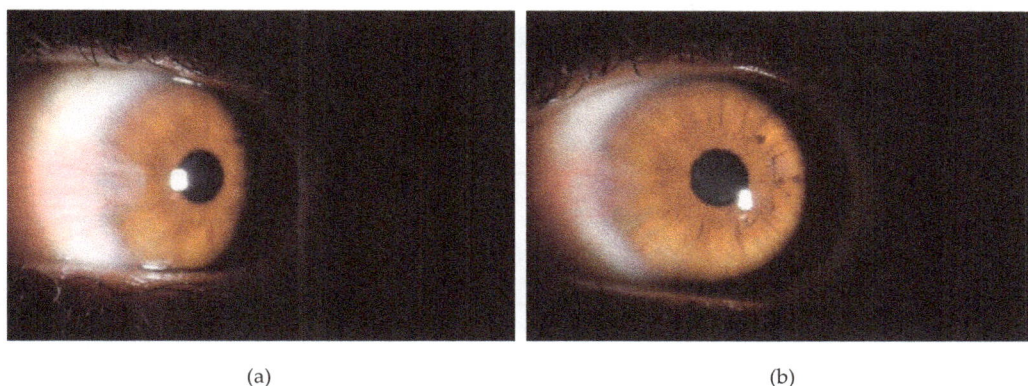

(a)   (b)

Figure 8. (a) Before MMC injection, (b) After MMC injection

All patients received one drop of chloramphenicol 0.5% and betamethasone 0.1% eye drops that were instilled four times daily for two days. After injection, patients were followed up at one day, one week, one month, six months, and one year. All patients were examined by a slit lamp at all visits for conjunctiva erythematic, epithelial defects, intraocular pressure, and other complications (complete slit-lamp examinations). The changes of pterygium size were evaluated by biomicroscope measurement (slit-lamp). (Base) × (apex) × (length) vs. mean size before and after MMC injection: (base means: up to down of pterygium in limbos, apex means: end of pterygium in cornea). The changes of refraction were also evaluated with topography and keratometer before and after injection.

Exclusion criteria were collagen vascular disease or other autoimmune diseases; pregnancy; ocular surface pathology or infectious, previous limbal surgery; and type III of pterygium.

3. Result

Of the 40 patients who participated in this study, 18 (45%) were males and 22(55%) were females. The mean age was 41.50 years. 16 (40%) left eye and 24 (60%) right eye. The patients were followed up from 12 to 14 months after injection (the mean follow-up period was 12 months). According to this study, 22.50% were farmers, 45% were housewives, and 32.50% had other occupations.

Within 1–3 days after the subconjunctival injection of MMC, 6 patients complained of irritation accompanied with mild conjunctiva swelling, hyperemia, and tearing (15%). These processes were controlled completely by using betamethasone 0.1% more frequently within 1 week. The pterygia were less vascular and less inflamed at the 6th-month visit after MMC injection.

We detected the reduced size of pterygium (mean size before MMC injection: 5.3mm (base) ×2.3 (apex) ×2.4(length) vs. mean size after MMC injection: 5mm (base) ×2.1mm (apex) ×1.56mm (length)) with mean 0.48 mm (base means: up to down of pterygium in limbos, apex means: end of pterygium in cornea that were evaluated by biomicroscope measurement (slit-lamp)). The size of pterygium was reduced in 83% of cases, and in all cases there were not seen progression and reduced the amount of astigmatism (mean 0.27 diopter) in 70% cases that were evaluated by topography and keratometry {p=0.00} (Table 2). We also detected no significant change in visual acuity and intraocular pressure.

	Sex		Job			Eyes		Age	
	Male	Female	Farmer	Housewives	Others	Left	Right	<40 years	>40 years
Number	18	22	9	18	13	16	24	16	24
Percent	45%	55%	22.50%	45%	32.50%	40%	60%	40%	60%
Total	40 100%			40 100%		40 100%		40 100%	

Table 1. The prevalence of study participant according to sex, job, age, and affected eye

	Hyperemia	Tearing	Long discomfort	Subconjunctival hemorrhage	pigmentation
1	+	+	-	-	-
2	+	+	+	-	-
3	-	+	+	-	-
4	+	-	+	-	-
5	+	+	+	+	-
6	+	-	-	-	-

Table 2. Dear Authors, please add Caption

	Before injection	After injection	P Value
Average of size pterygium	2.40	1.56	P=0.00
Average of refraction	1.19	0.92	P=0.00
Average of keratometry	1.67	1.33	P=0.00

Table 3. Complication of MMC injection in 6 patients

4. Discussion

Primary pterygium is one of the most common corneal disorders in topical countries such as India and south of Iran [4, 19]. A wide range of surgical procedures for removal of pterygia have been reported over the past decade, and several techniques are now available for the ophthalmic surgeon to choose from [4].

This study evaluated efficacy and complications of subconjunctival injection of MMC in treatment of primary pterygia. In fact, the potent effect of topical MMC on the conjunctiva epithelium has been demonstrated by its ability to prevent the recurrence of conjunctival intraepithelial neoplasia [14]. We use 0.1 ml of 0.2 mg/ml of MMC. Chen et al. [12] showed that a concentration of 0.10 mg/ml MMC inhibits fibroblast replication and that concentrations of 0.3 mg/ml actually cause death of fibroblasts.

Intraoperative use of MMC significantly retards epithelial healing in a dose-related manner in rabbit corneas [15]. In our study, 6 patients complained of irritation accompanied with mild conjunctiva swelling, hyperemia, and tearing (15%). These processes were controlled completely by using betamethasone 0.1% more frequently within one week. The pterygia were less inflamed at the 1st-month visit after MMC injection.

Recently, a new study evaluated adjunctive subconjunctival MMC (0.1 ml of 0.15 mg/ml) before pterygium excision. They reported recurrence rate of 6% with no sever complications [20, 21].

The advantage of low-dose subconjunctival MMC is that it is effective in preventing pterygium recurrence yet avoids the ocular surface toxicity associated with epithelial and bare sclera delivery of the medication. The medication is administered directly to the activated fibroblasts in the subconjunctival space, where it can work to avoid or diminish long-term epithelial healing difficulties associated with MMC. Intraoperative and postoperative MMC are two methods of adjunctive therapy that have been most commonly reported recently [22]. At the present time, we injected low dose subconjunctivally 0.1 ml of 0.2 mg/ml of MMC. Our short-term experience with MMC consistently shows no severe complications and reduces recurrence rate; these findings are similar to the study by Raiskup F et al. in 2004 [22]. Most of the complications of MMC are associated with persistent epithelial defects and ischemic sclera necrosis. Both of these complications are secondary to side effects produced by the direct action of MMC on these tissues. Because the epithelium and sclera are not target tissues for the MMC and because inadvertently treating these tissues does not contribute to the prevention of pterygia recurrence but is associated with significant side effects, the conjunctiva epithelium and sclera should be avoided. With subconjunctival application of MMC, the epithelial and sclera toxicity can be diminished; this occurred in our study. Eric D Donnenfeld et al reported that subconjunctival injection of MMC is an effective treatment before pterygium excision [23]. We chose their method but we used MMC in higher concentration (0.1 ml of 0.2 mg/ml) to reduce the size of pterygium.

In our study, the size of pterygium was reduced in 83% of cases and in all cases there were not seen progression and the amount of Astigmatism reduced (mean 0.27 diopter) in 70% cases that were evaluated by topography and keratometry (Table 1). In research by Khakshoor H et al, they found that subconjunctival injection of MMC reduced size and recurrence rate of pterygia [24]. Our study shows similar results. Also in another study, Oguz H, in Nassau University Medical Center, East Meadow, New York, USA [25], studied 36 eyes of 36 patients prospectively that received 0.1 ml of 0.15 mg/ml MMC subconjunctivally injected into the head of the pterygium 1 month before bare sclera surgical excision. He reported: the pterygia resolved in 34 (94%) of 36 eyes, with a recurrence rate of 6% over a mean follow-up of 24.4 months. No wound-healing complication developed in any patient. Their findings are similar to our study.

Therefore, low recurrence rate and safety profile with a mean follow-up of longer than 12 months without complication show the efficacy of this treatment and compare favorably with previous studies with MMC in the treatment of pterygia.

Limitation of the study: Despite the fact that we did not observe any significant short-term complications after MMC use, we are aware that only 40 patients were available for evaluation in our study.

We feel that adjunctive use of MMC for pterygium is a safe procedure, but requires a strict selection of patients, controlled use of MMC, and long-term follow-up of these patients. In particular, a very long follow-up of the avascular conjunctival area is required.

5. Conclusion

Subconjunctival injection of MMC is an effective treatment, and that is a promising alternative in the management of pterygium, but long-term follow-up is required.

Author details

Mohammad Hossien Davari[1,2], Hoda Gheytasi[3*] and Esmat Davari[1]

*Address all correspondence to: hoda24masoud @yahoo.com

1 Ophthalmology Department Vali e Asre Hospital, Birjand University of Medical Science, Birjand, Iran

2 Atherosclerosis and Coronary Artery Research Center, Birjand University of Medical Science, Birjand, Iran

3 Josep Font Laboratory of Autoimmune Disease, IDIBAPS, Hospital Clinic, Barcelona, Spain, Spain

References

[1] Cameron ME. Pterygium throughout the world. St. Louis: Mosby; 1965.

[2] Pang Y, Rose T. Rapid growth of pterygium after photorefractive keratectomy. Optometry. 2006; 77(10): 499-502.

[3] Sodhi PK, Verma L, Ratan SK. The treatment of pterygium. Surv Ophthalmol. 2004; 49 (5): 541-542.

[4] Panda A, Das GK, Tuli SW, Kumar A. Randomized trial of intraoperative mitomycin C in surgery for pterygium. Am J Ophthalmol. 1998; 125 (1): 59-63.

[5] Wan Norliza WM, Raihan IS, Azwa JA, Ibrahim M. Scleral melting 16 years after pterygium excision with topical Mitomycin C adjuvant therapy. Cont Lens Anterior Eye. 2006; 29 (4):165-167.

[6] Figueiredo RS, Cohen EJ, Gomes JA, Rapuano CJ, Laibson PR. Conjunctival autograft for pterygium surgery: how well does it prevent recurrence? Ophthalmic Surg Lasers. 1997; 28 (2): 99-104.

[7] Kenyon KR, Wagoner MD, Hettinger ME. Conjunctival autograft transplantation for advanced and recurrent pterygium. Ophthalmology. 1985; 92 (11): 1461-1470.

[8] Lewallen S. A randomized trial of conjunctival autografting for pterygium in the tropics. Ophthalmology. 1989; 96 (11): 1612-1614.

[9] Frucht-pery J, Raiskup F, Ilsar M, Landau D, Orucov F and Solomon A. Conjunctival autografting combined with low-dose mitomycin C for prevention of primary pterygium recurrence. Am J Ophthalmol. 2006; 141: 1044-1050.

[10] Gandolfi SA, Vecchi M, Braccio L. Decrease of intraocular pressure after subconjunctival injection of mitomycin in human glaucoma. Arch Ophthalmol. 1995; 113 (5): 582-585.

[11] Donnenfeld ED, Perry HD, Wallerstein A, Caronia RM, Kanellopoulos AJ, Sforza PD, et al. Subconjunctival mitomycin C for the treatment of ocular cicatricial pemphigoid. Ophthalmology. 1999; 106 (1): 72-78.

[12] Chen CW, Huang HT, Bair JS, Lee CC. Trabeculectomy with simultaneous topical application of mitomycin-C in refractory glaucoma. J Ocul Pharmacol. 1990; 6 (3): 175-182.

[13] Salomão DR, Mathers WD, Sutphin JE, Cuevas K, Folberg R. Cytologic changes in the conjunctiva mimicking malignancy after topical mitomycin C chemotherapy. Ophthalmology. 1999; 106 (9):1756-1760.

[14] Frucht-Pery J, Sugar J, Baum J, Sutphin JE, Pe'er J, Savir H, et al. Mitomycin C treatment for conjunctival-corneal intraepithelial neoplasia: a multicenter experience. Ophthalmology. 1997; 104 (12): 2085-2093.

[15] Ando H, Ido T, Kawai Y, Yamamoto T, Kitazawa Y. Inhibition of corneal epithelial wound healing. A comparative study of mitomycin C and 5-fluorouracil. Ophthalmology. 1992; 99 (12): 1809-1814.

[16] Rubinfeld RS, Pfister RR, Stein RM, Foster CS, Martin NF, Stoleru S, et al. Serious complications of topical mitomycin-C after pterygium surgery. Ophthalmology. 1992; 99 (11): 1647-1654.

[17] Mutlu FM, Sobaci G, Tatar T, Yildirim E. A comparative study of recurrent pterygium surgery: limbal conjunctival autograft transplantation versus mitomycin C with conjunctival flap. Ophthalmology. 1999; 106 (4): 817-821.

[18] Wong VA, Law FC. Use of mitomycin C with conjunctival autograft in pterygium surgery in Asian-Canadians. Ophthalmology. 1999; 106 (8): 1512-1515.

[19] Zanjani H, Nikandish M, Salari AM, Heyrani Moghadam H and Dashipoor A. Efficacy and safety of subconjunctival mitomycin C and Daunorubicin in the treatment of pterygium. Bina Ophthalmol. 2007; 12 (3): 367-372.

[20] Kee C, Pelzek CD, Kaufman PL. Mitomycin C suppresses aqueous human flow in cynomolgus monkeys. Arch Ophthalmol. 1995; 113 (2): 239-242.

[21] Lam DS, Wong AK, Fan DS, Chew S, Kwok PS, Tso MO. Intraoperative mitomycin C to prevent recurrence of pterygium after excision: a 30-month follow-up study. Ophthalmology. 1998; 105 (5): 901-904

[22] Raiskup F, Solomon A, Landau D, Ilsar M, Frucht-Pery J. Mitomycin C for pterygium: long term evaluation. Br J Ophthalmol. 2004; 88 (11): 1425-1428.

[23] Donnenfeld ED, Perry HD, Fromer S, Doshi S, Solomon R, Biser S. Subconjunctival mitomycin C as adjunctive therapy before pterygium excision. Ophthalmology. 2003; 110 (5): 1012-1016.

[24] Khakshoor H, Zarei S, Sharifi M, et al. Clinical result and complication of adjunctive subconjunctival mitomycin –C injection before pterygium excision. Iran J Ophthal. 2005; 18(2):70-6.

[25] Oguz H. Mitomycin C and pterygium excision,Ophthalmology. 2003 Nov; 110(11): 2257-2258.

Permissions

The contributors of this book come from diverse backgrounds, making this book a truly international effort. This book will bring forth new frontiers with its revolutionizing research information and detailed analysis of the nascent developments around the world.

We would like to thank all the contributing authors for lending their expertise to make the book truly unique. They have played a crucial role in the development of this book. Without their invaluable contributions this book wouldn't have been possible. They have made vital efforts to compile up to date information on the varied aspects of this subject to make this book a valuable addition to the collection of many professionals and students.

This book was conceptualized with the vision of imparting up-to-date information and advanced data in this field. To ensure the same, a matchless editorial board was set up. Every individual on the board went through rigorous rounds of assessment to prove their worth. After which they invested a large part of their time researching and compiling the most relevant data for our readers.

The editorial board has been involved in producing this book since its inception. They have spent rigorous hours researching and exploring the diverse topics which have resulted in the successful publishing of this book. They have passed on their knowledge of decades through this book. To expedite this challenging task, the publisher supported the team at every step. A small team of assistant editors was also appointed to further simplify the editing procedure and attain best results for the readers.

Apart from the editorial board, the designing team has also invested a significant amount of their time in understanding the subject and creating the most relevant covers. They scrutinized every image to scout for the most suitable representation of the subject and create an appropriate cover for the book.

The publishing team has been an ardent support to the editorial, designing and production team. Their endless efforts to recruit the best for this project, has resulted in the accomplishment of this book. They are a veteran in the field of academics and their pool of knowledge is as vast as their experience in printing. Their expertise and guidance has proved useful at every step. Their uncompromising quality standards have made this book an exceptional effort. Their encouragement from time to time has been an inspiration for everyone.

The publisher and the editorial board hope that this book will prove to be a valuable piece of knowledge for researchers, students, practitioners and scholars across the globe.

List of Contributors

Sanja Masnec and Miro Kalauz
Department of Ophthalmology, Zagreb University Hospital Centre, Zagreb, Croatia

Roy Schwartz and Zohar Habot-Wilner
Ophthalmology division, Tel-Aviv Medical Center, the Sackler Faculty of Medicine, Tel Aviv University, Israel

Miltiadis K. Tsilimbaris, Chrysanthi Tsika, George Kontadakis and Athanassios Giarmoukakis
University of Crete, Medical School, Department of Ophthalmology, Crete, Greece

César Hita-Antón
Department of Ophthalmology, Hospital Universitario de Torrejón, Torrejón de Ardoz, Madrid, Spain

Lourdes Jordano-Luna and Rosario Díez-Villalba
Department of Ophthalmology Hospital Universitario de Getafe, Getafe, Madrid, Spain
Universidad Europea de Madrid, Madrid, Spain

Patricia Durán Ospina and Mayra Catalina Cáceres Díaz
Visual Research Group Fundación Universitaria del Área Andina, Pereira, Colombia

Sabrina Lara
Universidad Nacional de Villa María, Córdoba, Argentina

Lik Thai Lim and Ahmed El-Amir
Dear Authors, please add affiliations, Country

Hiroshi Kobayashi
Department of Ophthalmology, Kanmon Medical Center, Shimonoseki, Japan

Dieudonne Kaimbo Wa Kaimbo
University of Kinshasa, Kinshasa, Congo (DRC)

Esmat Davari1
1 Ophthalmology Department Vali e Asre Hospital, Birjand University of Medical Science, Birjand, Iran

Mohammad Hossien Davari
Ophthalmology Department Vali e Asre Hospital, Birjand University of Medical Science Birjand, Iran Atherosclerosis and Coronary Artery Research Center, Birjand University of Medical Science, Birjand, Iran

Hoda Gheytasi
Josep Font Laboratory of Autoimmune Disease, IDIBAPS, Hospital Clinic, Barcelona, Spain

Index

www.ingramcontent.com/pod-product-compliance
Lightning Source LLC
Chambersburg PA
CBHW080642200326
41458CB00013B/4707